Mechanism of Artificial Heart

Takashi Yamane

# Mechanism of Artificial Heart

Springer

Takashi Yamane
School of Engineering, Kobe University
Kobe, Hyogo
Japan

ISBN 978-4-431-56705-9 ISBN 978-4-431-55831-6 (eBook)
DOI 10.1007/978-4-431-55831-6



Printed on acid-free paper

This Springer imprint is published by SpringerNature
The registered company is Springer Japan KK.

# Preface

As the author has been involved in medical engineering research at the National Institute of Advanced Industrial Science and Technology and also at Kobe University, in the development of a medical product with a company, and in regulatory affairs at the Pharmaceuticals and Medical Devices Agency, he thought that it would be useful to collect and record his knowledge. This book therefore describes design concepts for surgical blood pumps, so-called ventricular assist devices or mechanical circulatory supports, to assist blood circulation. Chapter 1 suggests medical care options to patients who need organ replacement or organ repair. Chapters 2, 3, 4, 5, 6, and 7 provide mainly the engineering tools including R&D and design evaluations. Chapter 8 describes bioreactions and evaluation methods. Among them, hemocompatibility refers to such factors as the reduction of blood cell/protein damage and the prevention of blood coagulation. In Chap. 9 it is shown how the devices are evaluated to verify their safety and efficacy for the purpose of clinical use. Finally, Chap. 10 describes the concluding remarks and future aspects.

Kobe, Japan　　　　Takashi Yamane

# Abbreviations

| | |
|---|---|
| AIAA | American Institute of Aeronautics and Astronautics |
| AIChE | American Institute of Chemical Engineers |
| ASAIO | American Society for Artificial Internal Organs |
| ASME | American Society of Mechanical Engineers |
| ASTM | American Society for Testing and Materials |
| FDA | U.S. Food and Drug Administration |
| ISO | International Organization for Standardization |
| JSAO | Japanese Society for Artificial Organs |
| METI | Ministry of Economy, Trade and Industry, Japan |
| MHLW | Ministry of Health, Labour and Welfare, Japan |
| NEDO | New Energy and Industrial Technology Development Organization, Japan |
| STS | Society of Thoracic Surgeons |

# Contents

# Chapter 1
# Introduction

Recent patients can choose a medical care among several opinions. Patients can choose medical care, medical device, regenerative medicine, or organ transplantation as long as it is ethical and donor organs/cells can be found. Especially patients, who received a diagnosis of necessity of organ replacement, will choose a care from mechanical artificial organs, regenerative tissues, or transplanted organs.

Organ transplantation is ideal because the patients can move or work without any restrictions after recover. For example, heart recipient can run after recover though his or her nerves are not connected to that of the donor heart. Transplantations are possible presently for heart, lung, kidney, pancreas, lever, intestine, and eyeball, the number of donors is limited (Fig. 1.1). Since a donor can provide seven organs, a donor patient can save seven recipient patients. However, the number of donors is limited in Asia. The number of donors is around 40 annually in Japan except for kidneys and eyeballs.

Artificial organs have been developed to replace the original organ functions even in emergency cases. Organs supporting high loadings and powers, such as artificial hearts, artificial lungs, artificial kidneys, artificial joints, and dental implants, have reached a practical use stage though artificial pancreas is still under a development stage (Fig. 1.1). Biomaterials for artificial skins, bones, artificial blood vessels, artificial or heart valves are available widely. For these organs, bioartificial organs, using cultured cells, are also under development.

Regenerative medicine will be able to replace or repair organ functions. Though autografts, namely self tissues, are thought to be safe for the patient, allografts, namely other person's tissues, can be applied widely if the immunity is suppressed (Fig. 1.1). The iPS cells can be applied to any patient without any rejections and can also be used to create new medicine against sick cells.

Now, serious heart patients can select options among emergency circulatory support, long-term implantable VAD, cell-sheets of heart muscle, and heart transplantation or their combinations.



T. Yamane, *Mechanism of Artificial Heart*, DOI 10.1007/978-4-431-55831-6_1

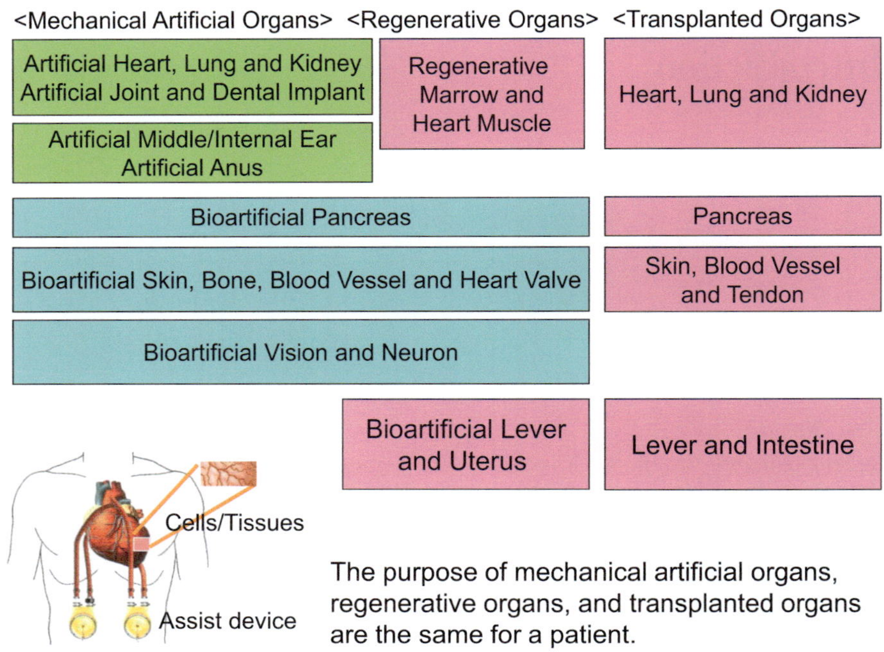


**Fig. 1.1** Organ replacement cares by mechanical artificial organs, regenerative organs, and transplanted organs

# Chapter 2
# What Kinds of Artificial Hearts Are Available?

## 2.1 Population of Heart Patients

The patient statistics in Japan is introduced first. 310,000 people died of cerebro-cardiovascular diseases annually. 300,000 patients are saved with physical treatment such as a stent therapy. 40,000 patients are saved with surgical operation using extracorporeal circulation. More than 400 patients are registered for heart transplantation at present and heart donors can be found less than 40 a year. Therefore roughly 260 or more patients should depend on ventricular assist devices. Actually ventricular assist devices are used for 140 patients a year.

## 2.2 Total-Replacement Artificial Hearts and Ventricular Assist Devices

Variations of the configurations of artificial hearts are shown in Fig. 2.1.

(1) Pneumatic driven pulsatile VAD for hospital use
(2) Pneumatic/hydraulic driven pulsatile VAD on a portable carry
(3) Electro-hydraulic total-replacement artificial heart (TAH)
(4) Implantable pulsatile VAD with electro-magnetic driver
(5) Implantable rotary VAD with mechanical bearings
(6) Implantable rotary VAD with non-contact bearings

The applicable pump mechanisms can be roughly classified into one with valves, one with rotary valves, and one without valves (Fig. 2.2). Using technical terms, they are

1. Pulsatile flow pump (Reciprocating pump): A type generating pulsatile flow by a reciprocating motion of a diaphragm with the aid of valves. Most of the early VADs were pulsatile flow pumps. Another pulsatile type drives flow through a



T. Yamane, *Mechanism of Artificial Heart*, DOI 10.1007/978-4-431-55831-6_2

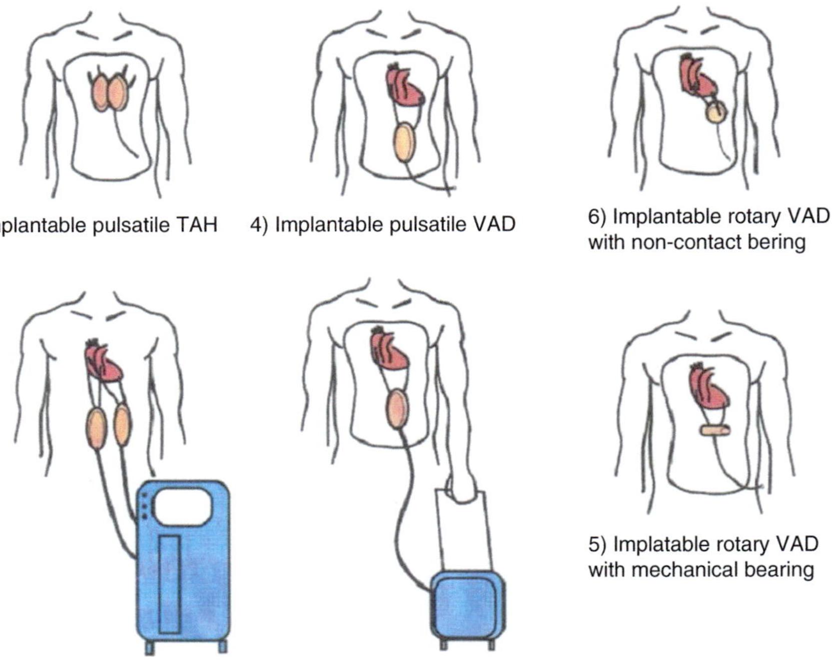


**Fig. 2.1** Classifications and configurations of artificial hearts

bucket relay with small compartments, which is sometimes called a rotary displacement pump. For example, a roller pump or a tube pump is used as a surgical pump.

2. Continuous flow pump (Rotary pump or Turbo pump): A type generating a continuous flow and a constant pressure with a constant rotational speed without valves. Most of the recent VADs are continuous flow pumps.

From a stand of clinical use, naming of pulsatile flow pumps and continuous flow pumps are often used to describe the blood flow characteristics.

Concrete pump configurations are listed in Fig. 2.2. For clinical use only a diaphragm pump, a pusher-plate pump, a roller pump, a centrifugal pump and an axial-flow pump have been applied so far.

A pulsatile flow pump drives a certain amount of blood with a stroke and determines flow rate, namely volume/time. On the other hand, a continuous flow pump generates a certain amount of pressure and the flow rate is determined by the body circulatory resistance, namely the patient's condition.

## 2.3 Generation Progress of Implantable Ventricular Assist Devices

The initial concept of an artificial heart was a total replacement of a natural heart since there was no extra space in the thorax surrounded by breast bones. It was called as a total-replacement artificial heart or a total artificial heart (TAH), which is

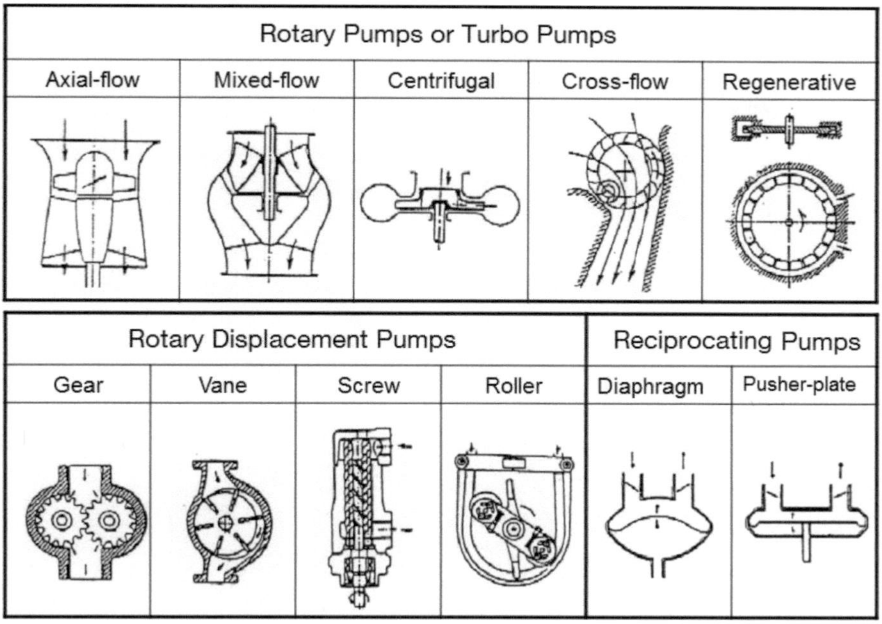


**Fig. 2.2** Classification of pump types

accompanied by removal of a natural heart. The first application to human was in 1969. The second use was a clinical trial of Jarvik-7 TAH in 1981 after the matuality of biocompatible materials. Though many total-replacement artificial hearts have been developed with pneumatic pulsatile mechanism, covering all of them is not the purpose of the present book. A landmark was thought to be the 'Abiocor' of an electro hydraulic pulsatile pump whose pump and energy transmitting coils were totally implanted. One of the presently available TAHs is SynCardia 'CardioWest', which was formally called 'Jarvik-7', and can now be used as temporary TAH (Fig. 2.3). Recent epoch making research is that two rotary pumps were used as a function of a total-replacement heart.

Then a new application preserving a natural heart and bypassing the left ventricle emerged, which is called a ventricular assist device (VAD). This type became recently a standard care for serious heart patients. Typical Japanese pulsatile VAD in-house use is Nipro VAD and is applied mainly before long-term implantable VADs (Fig. 2.3).

The progress of implantable VADs can be classified into three generations:

The first generation of implantable VAD was implantable pulsatile VADs with electro-magnetic driver, corresponding above item (4). Since their weight was more than 1 kg, they were applicable to patients who weigh more than 80 kg.

The second generation was brought by the emergence of rotary VADs with mechanical bearings, corresponding item (5). An innovation occurred in size of a blood pump and enabled patients to go out of hospital.

The third generation was brought by non-contact bearings, corresponding item (6). It extended dramatically the durability of VADs and enabled patients to return jobs and to use the VAD permanently.

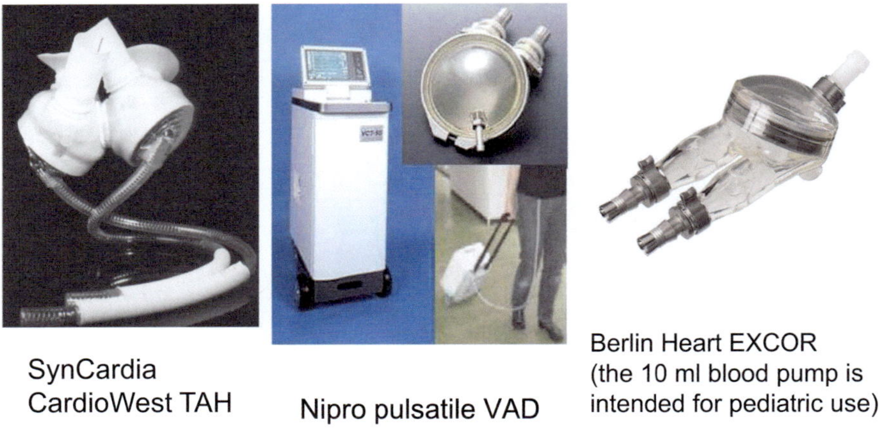


**Fig. 2.3** Pulsatile VAD/TAH for in-house use (Reproduced with permission of SynCardia Systems, Inc., Berlin Heart Inc., and Nipro Corp., respectively)

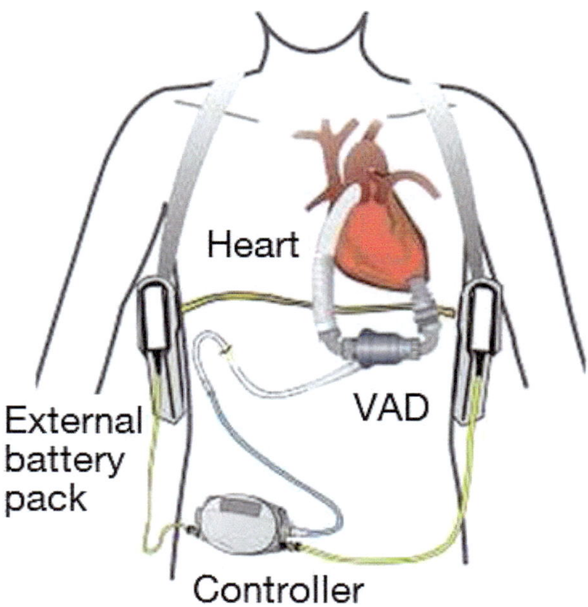


**Fig. 2.4** Recent configuration of an implantable VAD, example of HeartMate II (Reproduced with permission of Thoratec Corp.)

A typical configuration of presently available VADs is shown in Fig. 2.4. A ventricular assist system is composed mainly of a blood pump, a controller, and external batteries. A patient usually carries two batteries and charges other two batteries. Each battery can supply usually for more than 8 h.

## 2.4 Practical Artificial Hearts: 1st to 3rd Generation

A diaphragm type in hospital use is driven pneumatically and composed of blood pumps, a console, and blood/air tubes. It is driven through a polymer diaphragm by switching compressed air/vacuum. Typical devices are the Nipro VAD, the Abiomed AB5000, and the BerlinHeart EXCOR including pediatric use.

The first generation of implantable VADs consists of pulsatile pumps. A pusher plate type squeezes and expands a polymer sack with hard plates. WorldHeart 'Novacor' used a pusher plate with an electromagnet and Thoratec 'HeartMate XVE' with a ball screw (Fig. 2.5). Novacor was implanted to more than 1800 patients before 2008 and HearMate XVE to more than 4600 patients over the world. As a total-replacement heart (TAH), the Abiomed 'Abiocor' obtained FDA humanitarian device exemption (HDE) approval in 2006, which push/pulls blood through a polymer diaphragm using silicone oil, which is called an electrohydraulic type.

The second generation of VADs consists of implantable rotary pumps with mechanical bearings. Most of them are axial-flow-pumps such as the JarvikHeart 'Jarvik-2000', the Thoratec 'HeartMate-II', and the ReliantHeart 'HeartAssist 5' which was originally developed by NASA and Baylor College of Medicine (Fig. 2.6).

The third generation devices consist of implantable rotary VADs with non-contact bearings. Most of them are centrifugal-pumps such as the Terumo 'DuraHeart' using a magnetic bearing, the SunMedical 'EVAHEART' using hydrodynamic bearing/mechanical seal, and the HeartWare 'HVAD' using hydrodynamic bearing (Fig. 2.7). Axial flow pumps have also been developed such as BerlinHeart 'INCOR', and 'NEDO pump' though being in a development stage (Fig. 2.8).

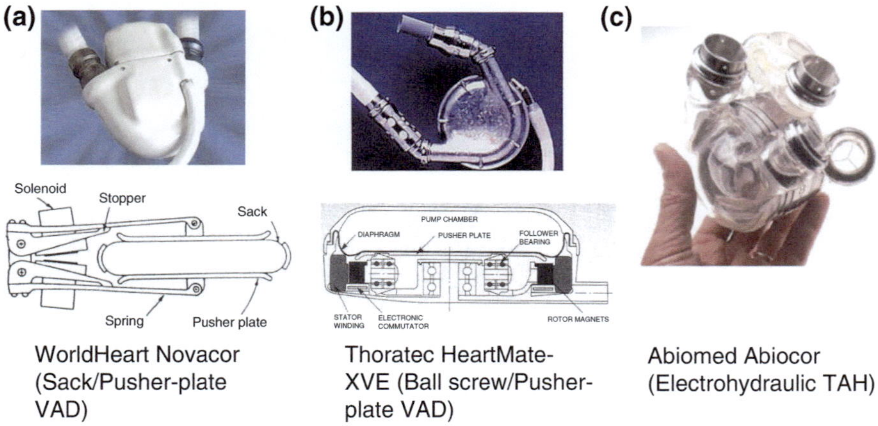


**Fig. 2.5** First generation of implantable VADs (Reproduced with permission of Thoratec Corp. and ABIOMED Inc., respectively)

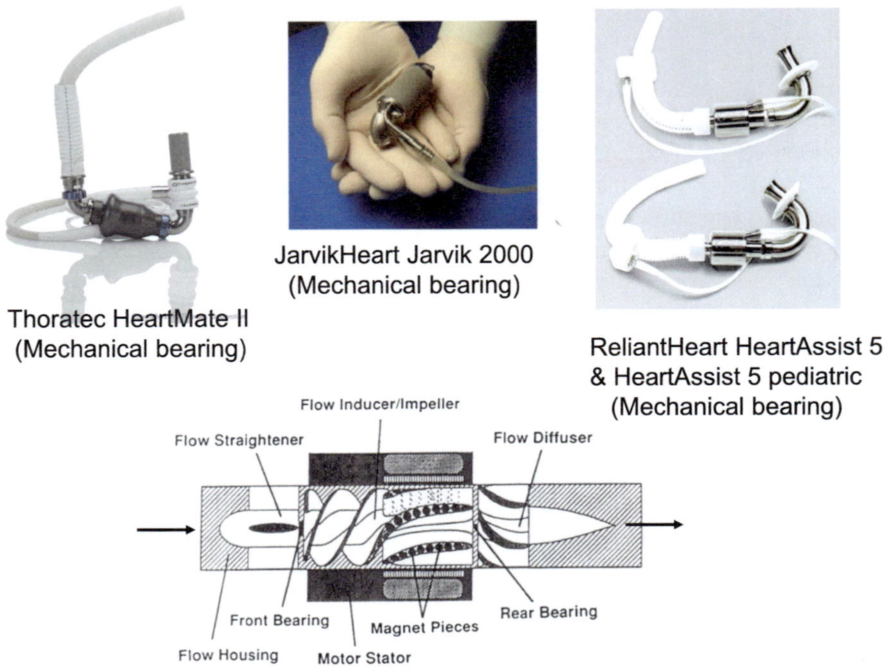


**Fig. 2.6** Second generation of implantable VADs; the structures are conceptual (Reproduced with permission of Wiley [1], Thoratec Corp., Jarvik Heart, Inc., and ReliantHeart Inc., respectively)

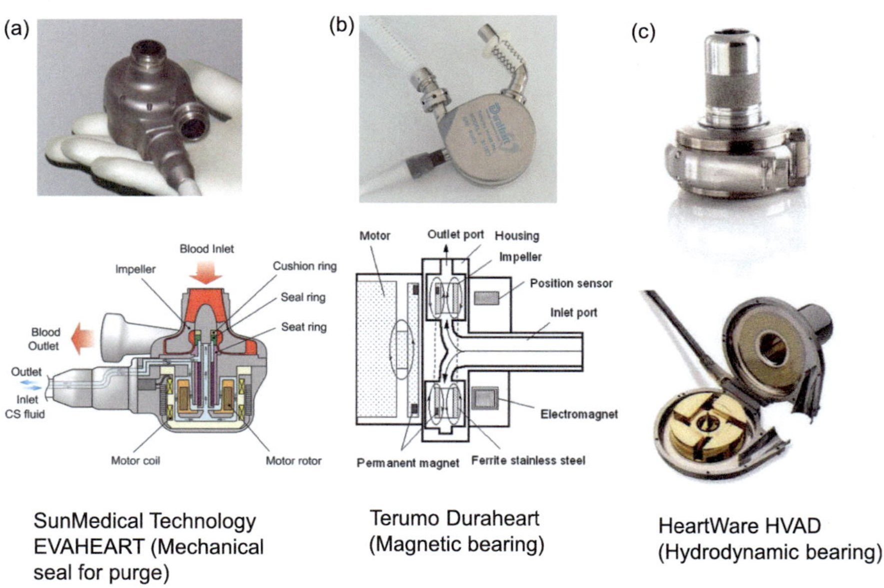


**Fig. 2.7** Third generation of implantable centrifugal VADs; the structures are conceptual (Reproduced with permission of Sun Medical Technology Research Corp., Tokyo Women's Medical University, Terumo Corp., and HearWare Inc., respectively)

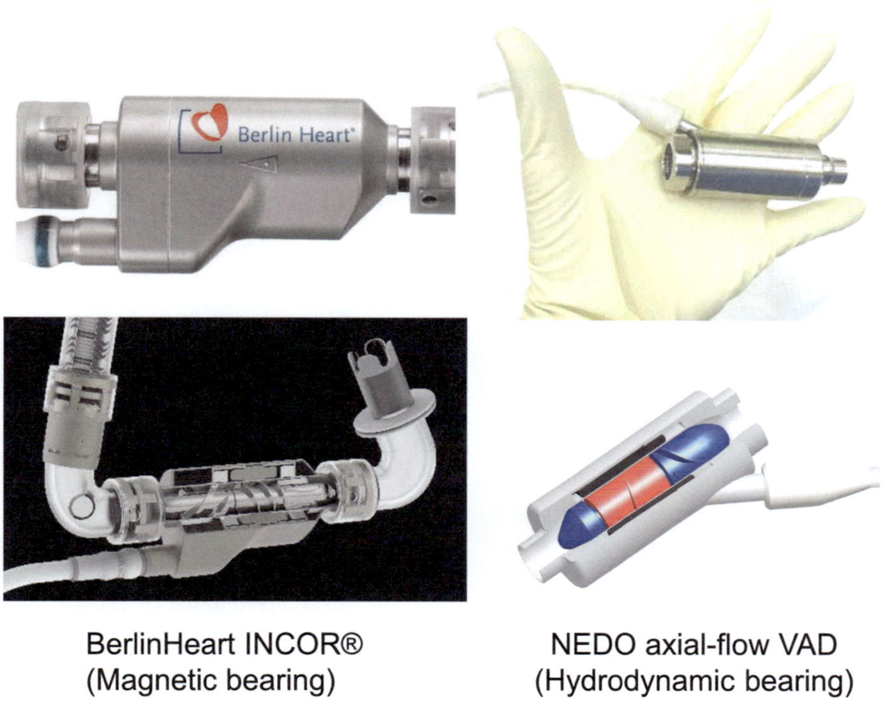


**Fig. 2.8** Third generation of implantable axial-flow VADs; the structures are conceptual (Reproduced with permission of Berlin Heart Inc. and NEDO, respectively)

Recently mechanical circulatory assist pumps have also become necessary for the term before VAD implantation. Thoratec ‘CentriMag’ conducted clinical trial as a short term VAD. Other candidates are emerging such as Maquet ‘Rotaflow’ or SenkoMedical ‘MERA centrifugal pump’ (Fig. 2.9). Recently, a small implantable pump are developed for a partial circulatory assist such as HeartWare ‘Synergy’. For emergency use, Abiomed ‘Impella’, a small axial flow pump, has been used like a balloon pump (Fig. 2.10).

A pump size comparison of VADs is shown in Fig. 2.11. It can be understand that recent implantable VADs weigh around 100 g though the early implantable VADs weigh more than 1000 g.

Clinical application of pulsatile flow and continuous flow VADs in the USA is shown in Fig. 2.12. In almost all cases, continuous flow VADs have been applied after 2010. They are used as bridge to transplantation (BTT) and bridge to candidacy (BTC), which means that an unqualified patient used VADs to improve his/her condition to qualification.

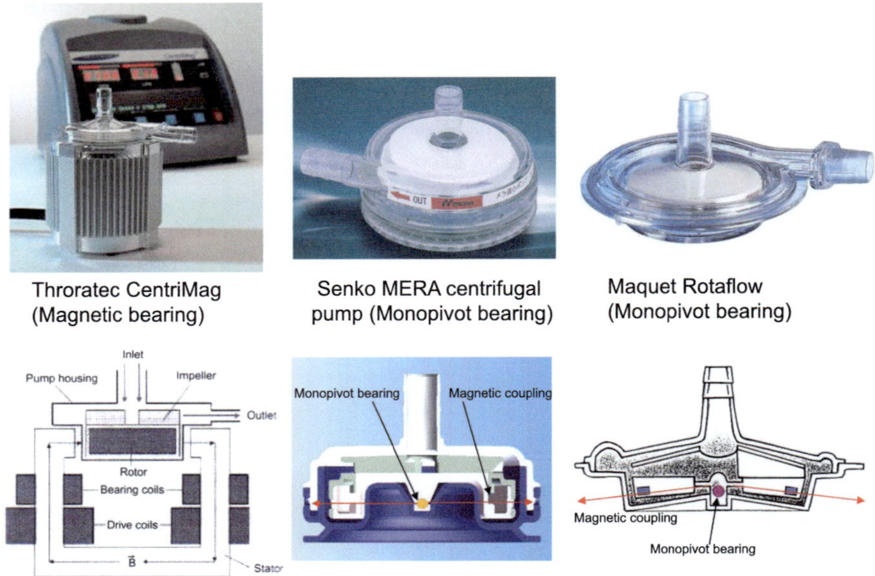


**Fig. 2.9** Mechanical circulatory assist pumps (Reproduced with permission of Thoratec Inc., Senko Medical Instrument Mfg. Co., Ltd., and Maquet Gettinge Group, respectively)

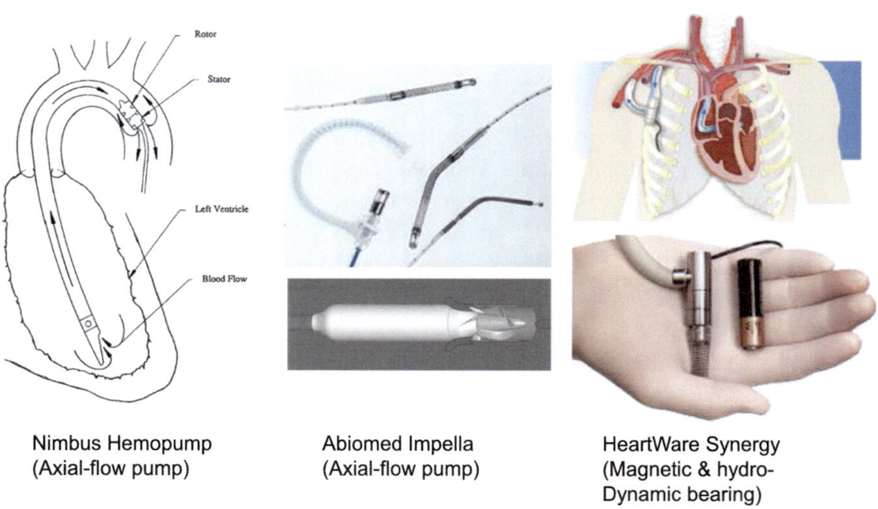


**Fig. 2.10** Mechanical circulatory assist pumps [2] (Reproduced with permission of ASAIO/ Walters Kluwer Health Inc., ABIOMED Inc., and HearWare Inc., respectively)

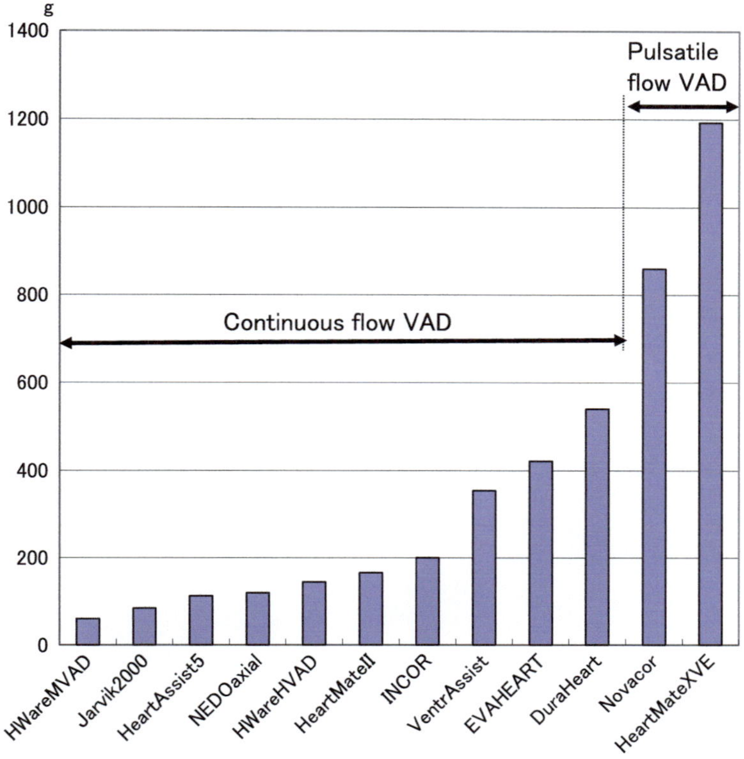


**Fig. 2.11** Pump size comparison of VADs

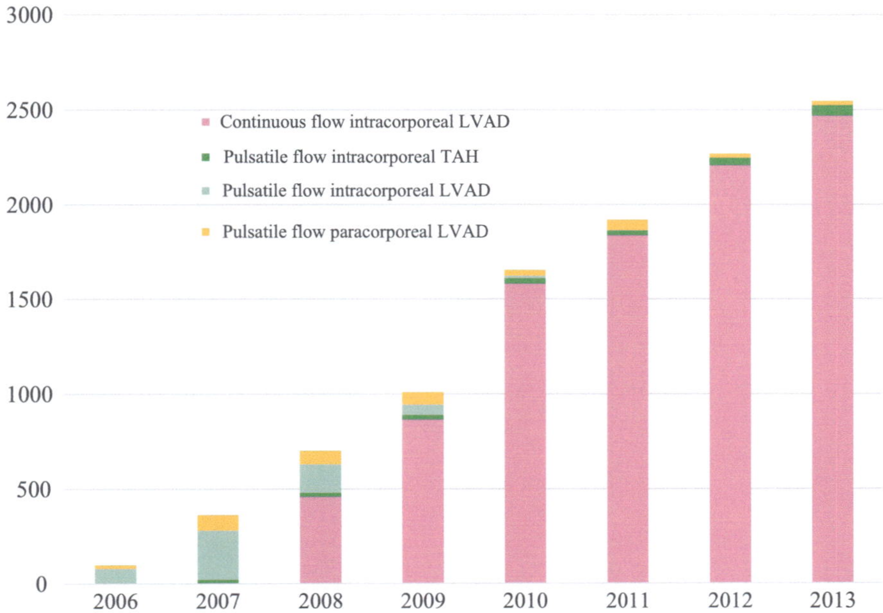


**Fig. 2.12** Tendency of clinical application of pulsatile-flow and continuous-flow VADs [3] (Implants data of INTERMACS 2006–2013, $N = 10542$)

## References

1. Mizuguchi, K., Damm, G., Benkowsky, R., Aber, G., Bacak, J., Svjkovsky, P., Glueck, J., Takatani, S., Nose, Y., Noon', G.P., DeBakey, M.E.: Development of an axial flow ventricular assist device: in vito and in vivo evaluation. Artif Organs, Blackwell **19**(7), 653–659 (1995)
2. Wampler, R.K., Moise, J.C., Frazier, O.H., Olsen, D.B.: In vivo evaluation of a peripheral vascular access axial flow blood pump. ASAIO Trans **34**, 450–454 (1988)
3. Kirklin, J.K., Naftel, D.C., Pagani, F.D., Kormos, R.L., Stevenson, L.W., Blume, E.D., Miller, M.A., Baldwin, J.T., Young, J.B.: Sixth INTERMACS annual report: a 10,000-patient database, InterMACS, Published Online: April 21, 2014 (2014)

# Chapter 3
# How Do We Select Pump Types?

## 3.1 Pulsatile Flow Pumps (Reciprocating Pumps and Rotary Displacement Pumps)

A pulsatile flow pump keeps a flow rate of a patient by driving a certain amount of blood, such as 70 mL, with a stroke. A sack type squeezes and expands a polymer sack pneumatically, namely by compressed/depressed air, or hydraulically, namely by silicone oil. A pusher plate type squeezes and expands a polymer sack with hard plates driven by an electromagnet or a motor/ball screw mechanism.

Since rotary displacement pumps, such as a roller pump or a tube pump, generate pulsatile flow, they are often classified as pulsatile flow pumps. In this type of pump, several rollers squeeze a tube and propel the blood forward. They have been used often in open heart surgery since only a tube is necessary for a patient.

## 3.2 Continuous Flow Pumps (Rotary Pumps or Turbo Pumps)

A "centrifugal pump" utilizes the outer pressure rise of a swirl (Fig. 3.1). As long as the rotational speed of swirl is maintained, it generates a certain pressure without regard to flow rate.

On the other hand, an "axial flow pump" changes the flow orientation by airfoils and obtains a pressure as a reaction force, which subsequently forms a swirl (Fig. 3.1). Since at a high flow rate the relative inflow angle becomes small, like a windmill, and a pressure becomes low and a higher rotational speed becomes necessary for high flow rates.

As long as the rotational speed of a rotary pump is maintained, a certain pressure rise is maintained even the external resistance, such as the aortic valve resistance, is changed. It results in the pulsatility of blood flow as shown in Fig. 3.2.



T. Yamane, *Mechanism of Artificial Heart*, DOI 10.1007/978-4-431-55831-6_3

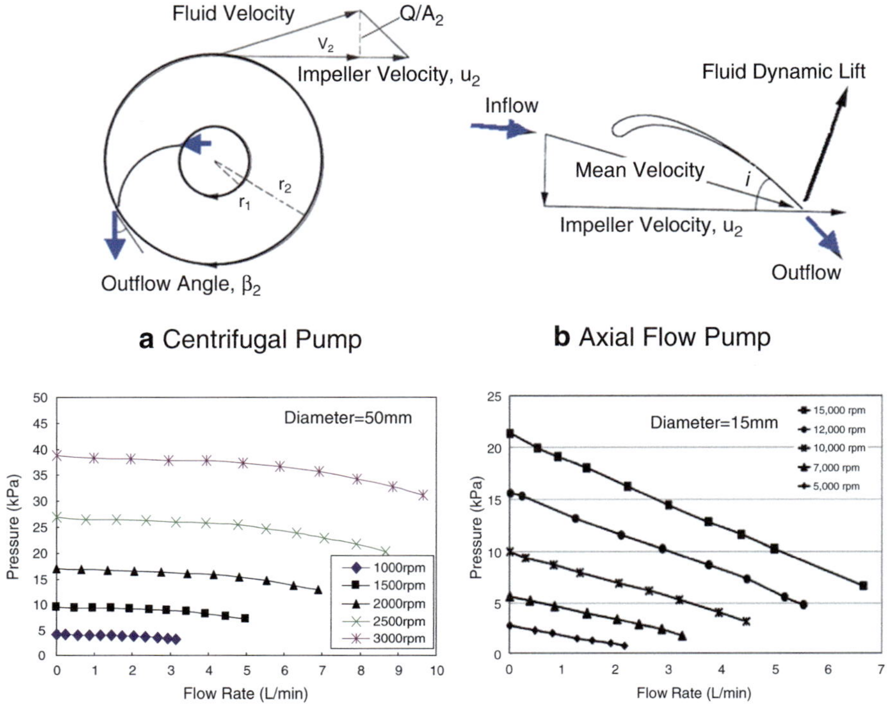


**Fig. 3.1** Centrifugal pump and axial flow pump

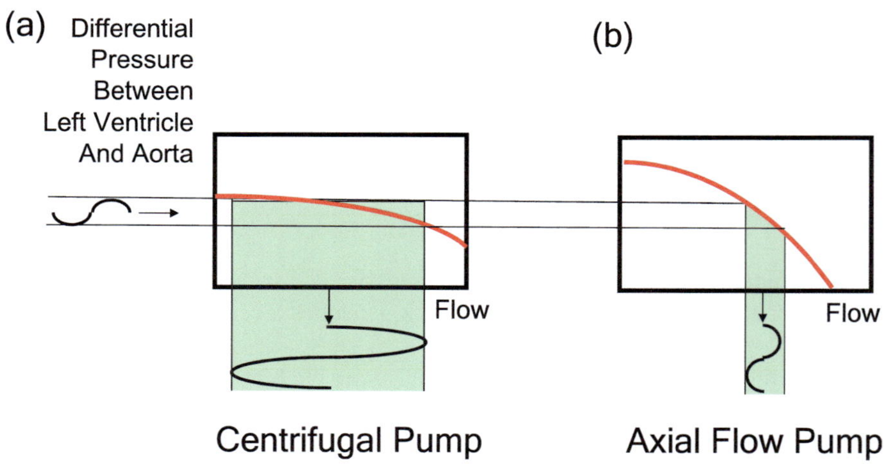


**Fig. 3.2** Pulsatility of rotary pumps

Though both types generate a pressure by making a swirl, there is a design continuity. The intermediate pump configuration between a centrifugal pump and an axial-flow pump is called “a mixed flow pump”. In the industrial pump designs, a

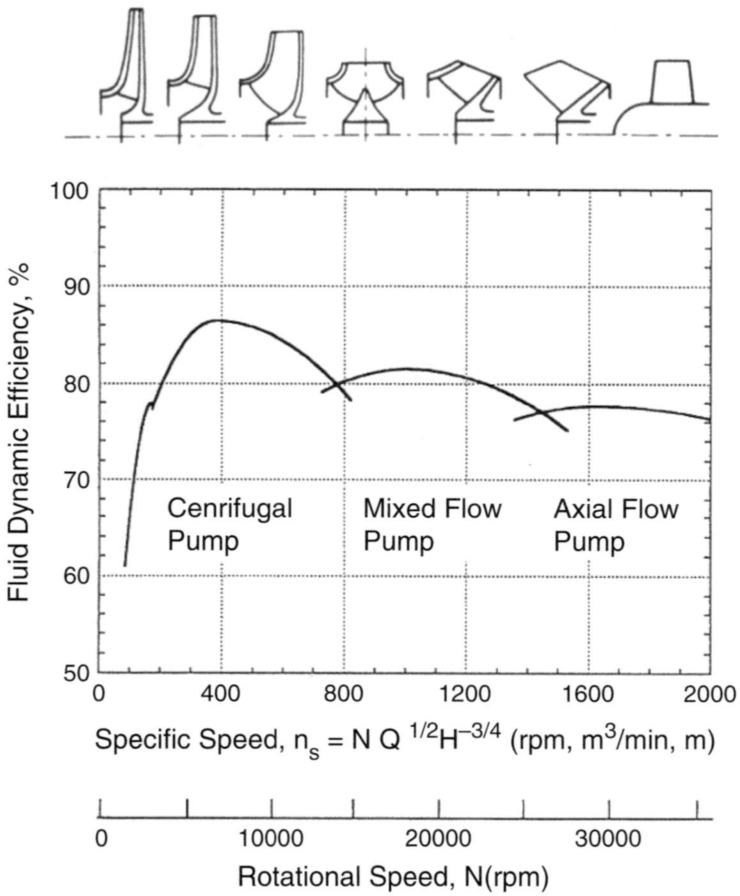


**Fig. 3.3** Selection of pump types

parameter named "specific speed" is often referred (Fig. 3.3). Specific speed is defined by

$$n_S \equiv \omega Q^{1/2} H^{-3/4}$$

where $\omega$ denotes angular velocity, $Q$ flow rate, and $H$ pressure head, respectively. When

$$gH = p/\rho = \eta(\omega R)^2$$

is inserted from pump theory using efficiency, $\eta$, *and gravity*, $g$,

$$n_S{}^2 = (g/\eta)^{3/2}(Q/R^2)/(\omega R)$$

Since $g/\eta$ is constant, it can be seen that the square of specific speed represents a ratio of [radial or axial velocity/tangential velocity]. The detail will be explained in the following section.

### *3.2.1 Pump Output*

The required performances to VAD pumps are as follows [1, 2]:

1. Mean pressure rise of 100 mmHg (80–120 mmHg) for left ventricular assist
2. Mean pressure rise of 20 mmHg (15–25 mmHg) for right ventricular assist
3. Mean blood flow rate of 5 L/min (2–10 L/min) for full support for an adult at a rest

Based on the turbo pump theory, the necessary torque to drive a pump, $T$, equals to the angular momentum change of fluid:

$$T = \rho Q(r_2 v_2 - r_1 v_1) \tag{3.1}$$

where $\rho$ *denotes* fluid density, $Q$ flow rate, $r$ radius, $v$ fluid rotational velocity, $(\ )_1$ inlet position, and $(\ )_2$ outlet position. Strictly speaking for an axial flow pump,

$$T = \rho \int_0^R \frac{\mathrm{d}Q'}{\mathrm{d}r}\left(v_2'(r) - v_1'(r)\right) r\mathrm{d}r,$$

This equation can be unified into Eq. (3.1), when a typical radius, $r_m$, is introduced as

$$T = \rho Q r_m (v_2 - v_1); \quad r_m = \frac{1}{Q}\int_0^R \frac{\mathrm{d}Q'}{\mathrm{d}r} \frac{\left(v_2'(r) - v_1'(r)\right)}{v_2 - v_1} r\mathrm{d}r$$

The present approximation holds only for pumps with small vane height such as VAD pumps. The input work and output work can be connected with fluid dynamic efficiency, $\eta$ as:

$$\eta\omega T = \Delta P \cdot Q$$

where $\omega$ denotes impeller rotational speed and $\Delta P$ differential pressure, which is, strictly speaking, a total pressure rise of fluid. Therefore $\Delta P$ can be derived as:

$$\Delta P/\rho = \eta(u_2 v_2 - u_1 v_1), \text{ where } u_1 = \omega r_1, u_2 = \omega r_2.$$

If there is no pre-rotation, namely $u_1 = 0$, then it becomes simply as

$$\Delta P/\rho = \eta u_2 v_2.$$

This means that the obtained pressure is proportional to the fluid circumferential velocity, $v_2$, at a constant rotational speed, $u_2$, and that the obtained pressure is proportional to $u_2^2 = r_2^2 \omega^2$ at a constant flow rate. It is important that this equation is valid not only for centrifugal pumps but also for axial-flow pumps. Therefore, [radius] × [rotational speed] is an important design parameter and defines a design limitation if the pump pressure is given (Fig. 3.4). When the pressure rise of 13.3 kPa (100 mmHg) is required, at least rotational velocity of 3.7 m/s is necessary for centrifugal pump and that of 5.2 m/s for an axial flow pump.

For a centrifugal pump, the fluid circumferential velocity, $v_2$, can be calculated with Fig. 3.1 as follows:

$$v_2 = u_2 - \frac{Q}{A_2} \frac{1}{tan\beta_2}$$

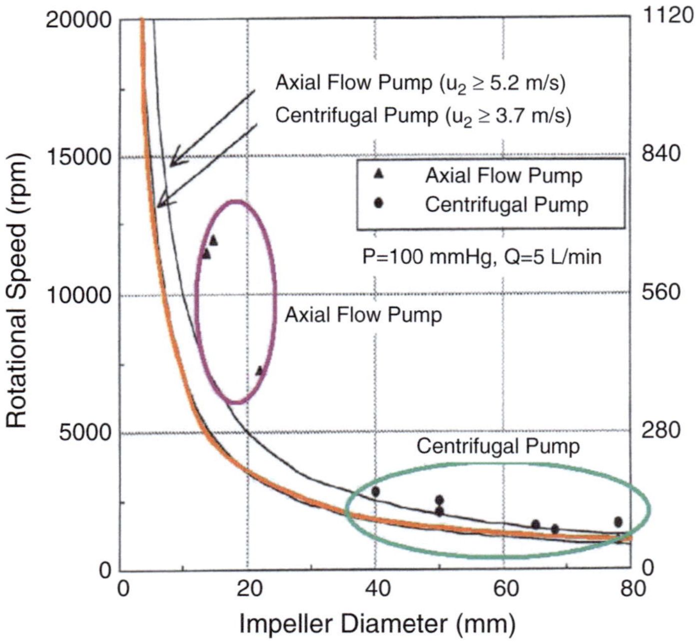


**Fig. 3.4** Design parameters of centrifugal pumps and axial flow pumps

where $A_2$ and $\beta_2$ are section area and outflow angle at the tip of the centrifugal impeller. This implies that the circumferential velocity, $v_2$, is almost equal to the impeller rotational velocity, $u_2$, as long as outflow angle, $\beta_2$, is nearly equal to 90°.

Regarding an axial-flow pump, based on Kutta-Joukowsky's theorem, a lift generated by an airfoil, $L$, is described by

$$L = \frac{1}{2}\rho c_m W^2 C_L = \rho W \Gamma; \quad \Gamma = v_2 \frac{2\pi r_m}{b}$$

where $W$ denotes mean relative velocity, $C_L$ lift coefficient, $c_m$ blade chord length, $r_m$ typical radius, and $b$ number of blades, respectively. Then, the fluid circumferential velocity, $v_2$, can be written with Fig. 3.1 as follows:

$$v_2 = \frac{1}{2}\sigma_m C_L W; \quad \sigma_m = \frac{bc_m}{2\pi r_m}; \quad W^2 = (u_2)^2 + \left(\frac{Q}{A_2}\right)^2$$

where $A_2$ denotes flow section area. The above lift coefficient, $C_L$, can be estimated with airfoil incident angle, $i$, and flow rate, $Q$, by

$$C_L = \frac{\mathrm{d}C_L}{\mathrm{d}\alpha}\alpha \cong 5.73\alpha; \quad \alpha = i - tan^{-1}\frac{Q}{A_2 u_2}$$

This implies that when the flow rate, $Q$, increases, the relative angle, $\alpha$, decreases and then the circumferential velocity, $v_2$, as well as the pump pressure, $\Delta P$, decreases until they reach zero.

### 3.2.2 Volute and Diffuser

Fundamental concept of fluid dynamic design of a continuous flow pump is that we should keep the flow velocity as constant as possible not to cause fluid dynamic loss, which can be attained by continuous section area distribution. Only at the vane area, the perpendicular velocity components are independently designed to obtain centrifugal pressure and tangential velocity. The total pressure rise is composed of static pressure rise and tangential velocity increase. The latter, high tangential velocity, can be changed to pressure at the so-called diffuser by expanding section area and reducing the velocity as is shown in Fig. 3.5. On the other hand, just collecting flow at the end of impeller without change of pressure is called volute, which corresponds to spiral shape as is shown in Fig. 3.5.

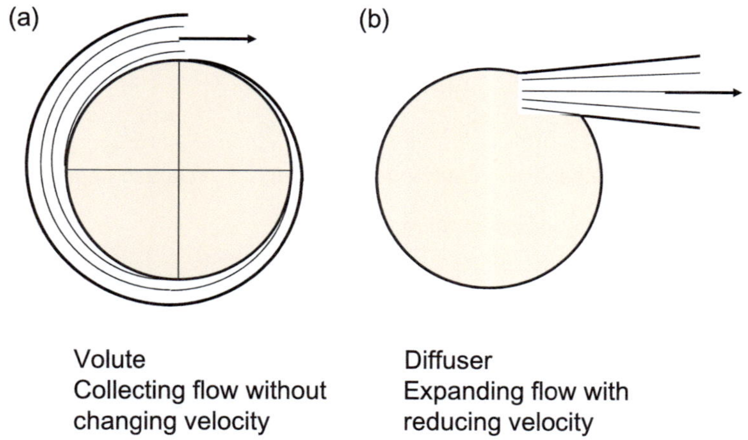


**Fig. 3.5** Volute and diffuser

### *3.2.3 Force Balance of a Centrifugal Impeller*

To obtain the static pressure distribution in the impeller plane for a centrifugal pump the equation of motion in cylindrical coordinates without external forces is used:

$$\frac{\partial u}{\partial t}+u\frac{\partial u}{\partial r}+\frac{v}{r}\frac{\partial u}{\partial \theta}+w\frac{\partial u}{\partial z}-\frac{v^2}{r}=-\frac{1}{\rho}\frac{\partial p}{\partial r}$$

Neglecting the variation with respect to $t$, $z$, and $\theta$, it becomes

$$u\frac{\partial u}{\partial r}-\frac{v^2}{r}=-\frac{1}{\rho}\frac{\partial p}{\partial r}$$

We assume a solid rotation with angular velocity $\omega$ and neglect the radial velocity $u$ for simplicity,

$$\frac{1}{\rho}\frac{\partial p}{\partial r}=r\omega^2; \quad v=r\omega$$

Then the static pressure in the impeller plane becomes a parabolic distribution as follows:

$$p(r)=\frac{1}{2}\rho\omega^2r^2+p_0 \tag{3.2}$$

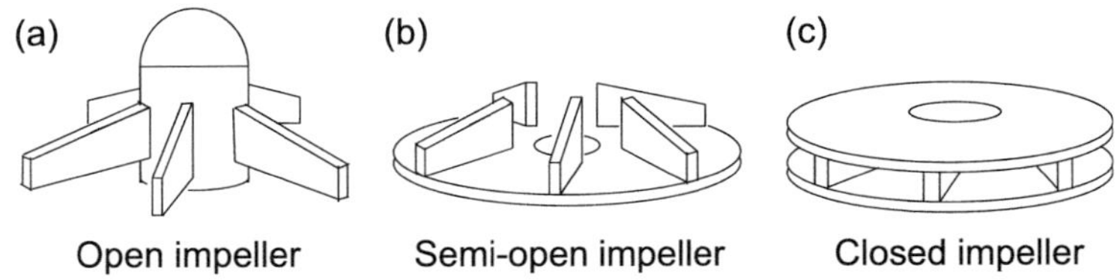


**Fig. 3.6** Open, semi-open, and closed type impellers

### *3.2.4 Open, Semi-Open, and Closed Type Impellers*

There are three ways of designing axial force balance of a centrifugal impeller by selecting shroud disks covering vanes.

When both sides of vanes are covered by two disks, or shrouds, it is called a 'closed-type impeller' (Fig. 3.6). The axial force equals to the difference between the upper gap and the lower gap. Since the pressure distributions, from the vane tip pressure to the central inlet pressure, are almost the same in both gaps, the axial force is small for a closed-type impeller. The fluid dynamic friction loss, however, is a little higher than other types.

When a side of vanes is covered by a disk, or a shroud, it is called a 'semi-open-type impeller'. The upper side pressure is shown as Eq. (3.2), and the bottom side pressure is almost the same as the vane tip pressure and reaches to the inlet pressure at the center. Therefore a semi-open-type impeller sometimes produces a large axial force. If the bottom side pressure is approximated as the vane tip pressure, namely the pressure difference is assumed as

$$\Delta p(x) = \left(1 - x^2\right) \times 13 \ \text{kPa}; \quad x = r/R$$

the maximum lifting force, $A\int \Delta p(x) x dx$, would be around

$$20 \ \text{cm}^2 \times 13 \ \text{kPa} \times (1 - 2/4) = 13 \ \text{N} \cong 1300 \ \text{gf}$$

When no shroud disks exist, it is called an 'open impeller'. Since the pressure distribution is shown as Eq. (3.2), which is common from top to bottom, the axial force is small for an open-type impeller. The fluid dynamic friction loss is the minimum among the three types.

### *3.2.5 Force Balance of an Axial-Flow Impeller*

On the other hand, axial-flow impeller supports the difference pressure of the inlet and outlet by the small disk area such as 1 cm$^2$. Then the axial force would be only

$$13\ \text{kPa} \times 1\ \text{cm}^2 = 1.3\ \text{N} \cong 130\ \text{gf}.$$

This can reduce the axial wear of bearing and can enhance the durability.

## References

1. Yamane, T., Ikeda, T.: Toyoki Orita and Tetsuya Tateishi: fluid dynamics of turbo pumps for artificial hearts. Mater. Sci. Eng. C **4**(2), 99–106 (1996)
2. Stepanoff, A.J.: Centrifugal and Axial Flow Pumps, 2nd edn. Krieger, Malabar (1993)

# Chapter 4
# Selection of Bearing Types: A Key to Durability

## 4.1 Pivot Bearing

The second generation implantable VADs are mostly axial flow pumps whose impellers are supported with mechanical bearings, especially with pivot bearings (Fig. 4.1). The typical VADs are the JarvikHeart 'Jarvik-2000', the Thoratec 'HeartMate-II', and the ReliantHeart 'HeartAssist 5'. In the field of extracorporeal centrifugal pumps, such as Maquet 'Rotaflow' or Senko Medical 'MERA centrifugal pump' [1], their impellers are supported with a single pivot, which is a so-called monopivot bearing.

For a pivot bearing, the wear, hemolysis, and thrombus formation at the pivot should be avoided. In a case of axial magnetic flux coupling, Dr. O. Maruyama showed experimentally the hemolysis depends on the contact areas using a monopivot centrifugal pump (Fig. 4.2). In a case of radial magnetic flux coupling, we recently found the hemolysis was not so dependent to contact areas using a centrifugal pump without vanes or an outlet (Fig. 4.3). The hemolysis index, NIH, is roughly a time gradient of plasma free hemoglobin, whose detail will be discussed later. Though these results showed a contrast, we should consider simultaneously the effect of magnetic forces.

On the other hand, how to reduce the rotational wear will be discussed in the chapter of bearing material and the improvement of thrombus formation in the chapter of in vitro anti-thrombogenicity test.

## 4.2 Magnetic Bearing and Hydrodynamic Bearing

The third generation implantable VADs are mostly centrifugal pumps with non-contact bearings. There are two types for non-contact bearings: one is a magnetic bearing and the other is a hydrodynamic bearing (Fig. 4.1).



T. Yamane, *Mechanism of Artificial Heart*, DOI 10.1007/978-4-431-55831-6_4

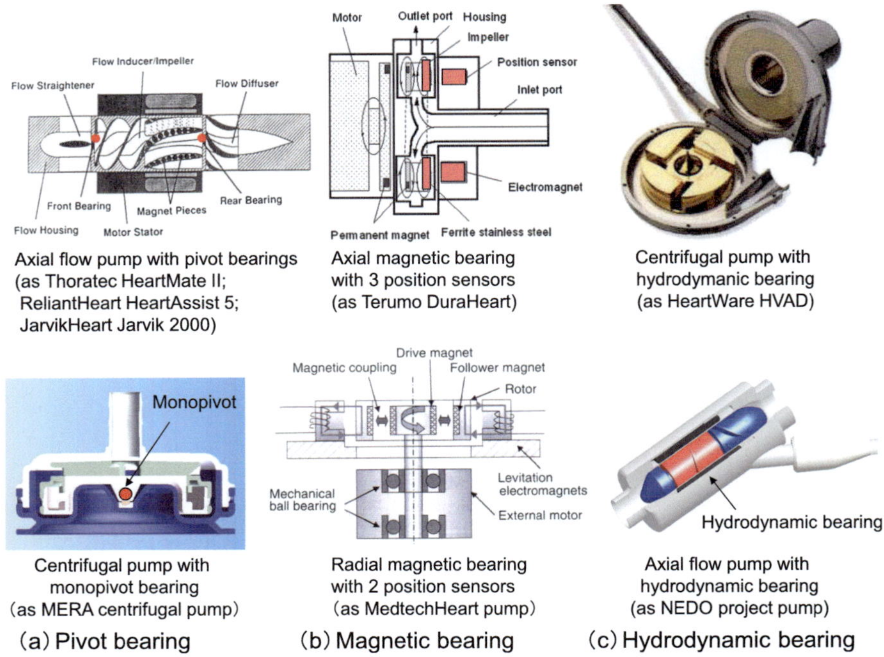


**Fig. 4.1** Classification of bearing types (Reproduced with permission of Wiley [2], ReliantHeart Inc., Senko Medical Instrument Mfg. Co., Ltd., Terumo Corp., MedtechHeart, Inc., HeartWare Inc., and NEDO, respectively)

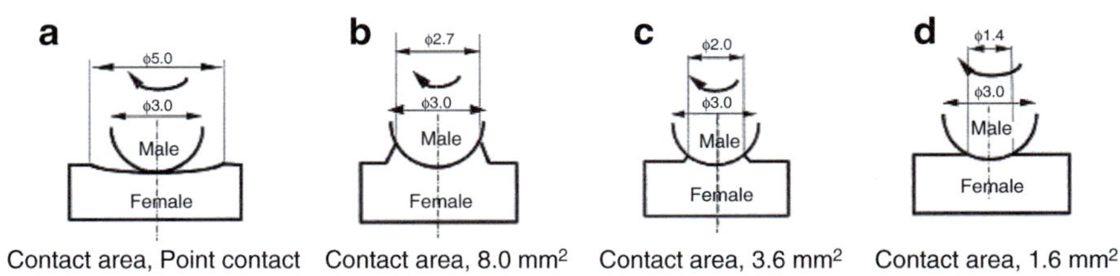


Hemolysis index, NIH, of centrifugal pumps (g/100L)

| Pivot Shape | NIH of each test pump | NIH of a commercial centrifugal pump | Relative index |
|---|---|---|---|
| a | 0.001 | 0.003 | 0.3 |
| b | 0.010 | 0.003 | 3.3 |
| c | 0.012 | 0.004 | 3.0 |
| d | 0.002 | 0.002 | 1.0 |

**Fig. 4.2** Effect of contact area of pivot bearings on hemolysis for a centrifugal pump with an axial flux coupling [3]

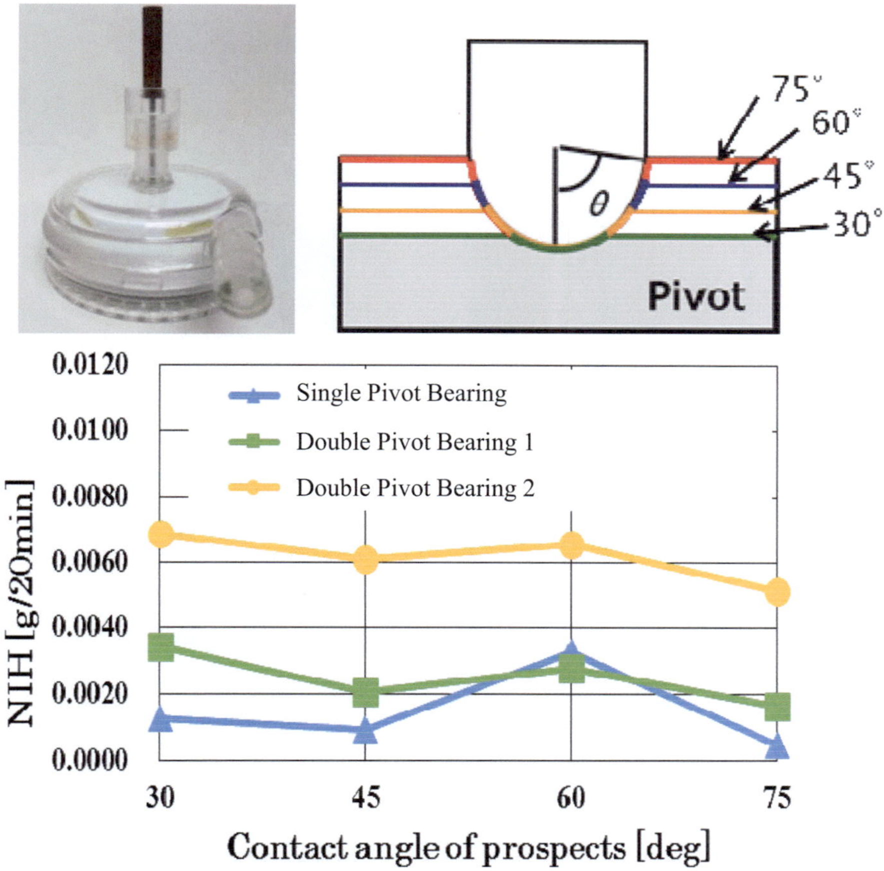


**Fig. 4.3** Effect of contact area of pivot bearings on hemolysis for a centrifugal pump with a radial flux coupling [4]

The magnetic bearing is composed of stator coils and position sensors to maintain the rotor at a position. If the position sensor is axial, three sensors are necessary to maintain a rotating plane. If the position sensor is radial and the axial position is maintained by magnets, only two sensors are necessary to maintain the rotor at the center, as shown in Fig. 4.1b. The motor mechanism is generally implemented separately.

The hydrodynamic bearing utilizes locally high pressures generated by fluid squeezed into a wedge-shaped channel or a step channel composed of relatively moving surfaces. An example of hydrodynamic bearing design is shown in Fig. 4.4.

As mentioned, the third generation devices consist of implantable rotary VADs with non-contact bearings. The Terumo 'DuraHeart' utilizes a magnetic bearing on the front side and a motor on the rear side. The SunMedical 'EVAHEART' utilizes a mechanical seal, separating blood and water with a submicron water film, and also

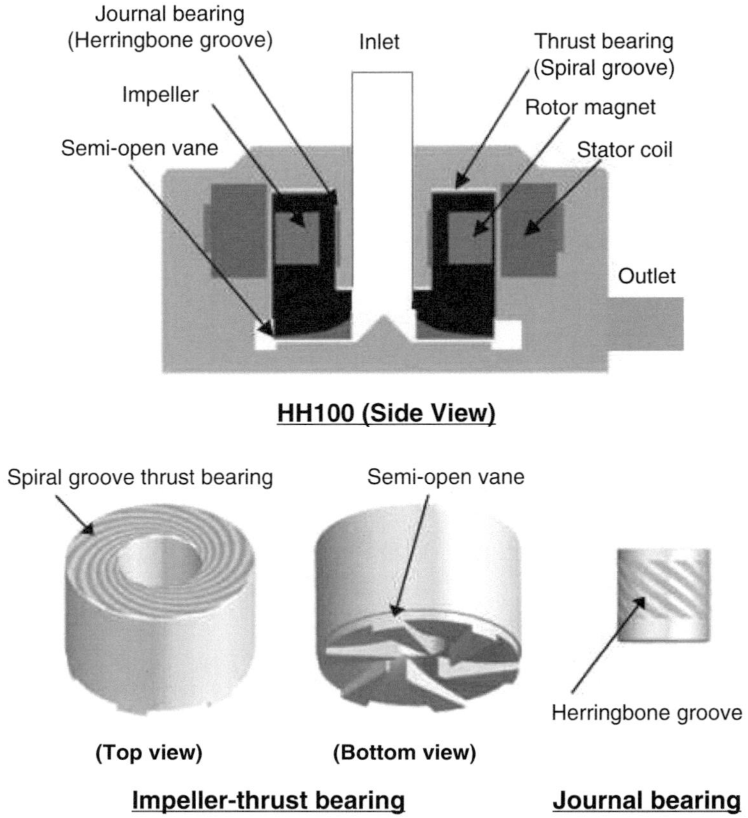


**Fig. 4.4** A design example of a hydrodynamic bearing pump [5]

a hydrodynamic bearing for motor axis. The HeartWare 'HVAD' utilizes hydrodynamic bearings and with magnetic suspension.

As bridge-to-decision devices, high-performance rotary pumps have also emerged. Among them is a magnetic-bearing centrifugal pump, the Thoratec 'CentriMag', which can be used over several months.

## 4.3 Analysis of Hydrodynamic Bearing

To analyze hydrodynamic bearings Reynolds equation in lubrication is useful and will be explained below [6].

When the gap size of bearing is denoted by $h(x, y)$, pressure by $p(x, y)$, and viscosity by $\mu$, the two-dimensional Reynolds equation in lubrication is described as follows:

$$\frac{\partial}{\partial x}\left(h^3\frac{\partial p}{\partial x}\right)+\frac{\partial}{\partial y}\left(h^3\frac{\partial p}{\partial y}\right)=6\mu\frac{\partial}{\partial x}(hU)$$

When the geometric depth distribution $h(x, y)$ and the boundary conditions are given, the pressure distribution $p(x, y)$ can be obtained over the gap surface of the bearing. When the system is one-dimensional, neglecting $y$ variation and the slope of the gap is linear, the solution becomes as

$$p=\frac{6\mu UL}{h^2}\frac{(h_1-h)(h-h_2)}{{h_1}^2-{h_2}^2}$$

This implies that the pressure is positive, $p > 0$, if $h_1 > h > h_2$, and that the pressure $p$ is proportional to the velocity $U$ and the length $L$ and inversely proportional to $h^2$. Two examples follow.

1. When a linear slope geometry is assumed as

$$h(x)=h_1-(h_1-h_2)\frac{x}{L};\quad h_1>h_2$$

Then the corresponding pressure distribution becomes (Fig. 4.5a)

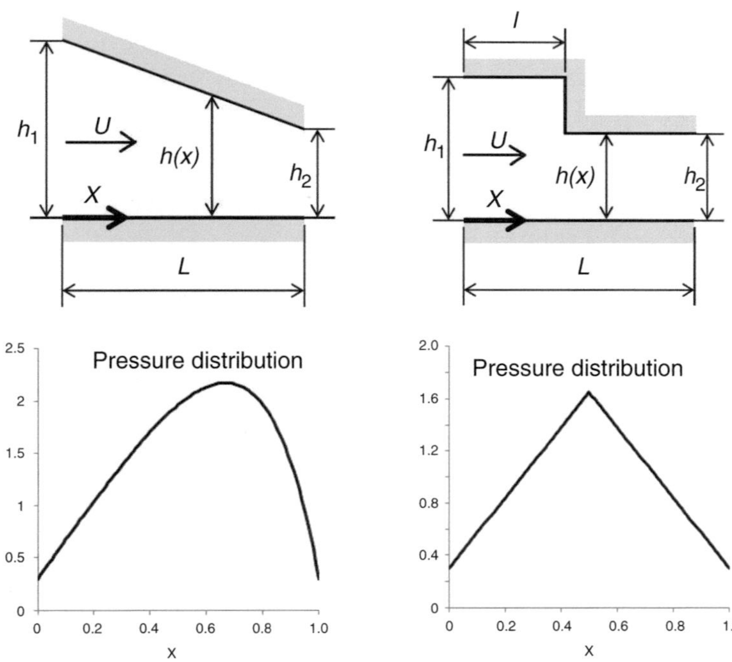


**Fig. 4.5** Pressure distribution of hydrodynamic bearing for different configurations: (**a**) a linear slope type and (**b**) a step type

$$p(x) = p_0 + 6\mu U \frac{L}{{h_1}^2 - {h_2}^2} \frac{x(L-x)}{(x-e)^2}; \quad e = \frac{h_1 L}{h_1 - h_2}$$

2. When a step geometry is assumed as

$$\begin{aligned} h &= h_1 \quad (0 \le x \le d) \\ h &= h_2 \quad (d \le x \le L); \quad h_1 > h_2 \end{aligned}$$

Then the corresponding pressure distribution becomes (Fig. 4.5b)

$$\begin{aligned} p(x) &= p_0 + 6\mu U \frac{(h_1 - h_2)(L-d)x}{(L-d){h_1}^3 + d{h_2}^3} \quad (0 \le x \le d) \\ p(x) &= p_0 + 6\mu U \frac{(h_1 - h_2)d(L-x)}{(L-d){h_1}^3 + d{h_2}^3} \quad (d \le x \le L) \end{aligned}$$

The detail to analyze the pressure distribution for the hydrodynamic bearing is shown below.

Velocities along $x$, $y$, $z$ are denoted by $u$, $v$, $w$. time by $t$, pressure by $p$, viscosity by $\mu$, and density by $\rho$. $\mu$ and $\rho$ are regarded as constants here.

Navier-Stokes equations are as follows:

$$x\text{-direction}: \rho\left(\frac{\partial u}{\partial t} + u\frac{\partial u}{\partial x} + v\frac{\partial u}{\partial y} + w\frac{\partial u}{\partial z}\right) = -\frac{\partial p}{\partial x} + \mu\left(\frac{\partial^2 u}{\partial x^2} + \frac{\partial^2 u}{\partial y^2} + \frac{\partial^2 u}{\partial z^2}\right) \tag{4.1}$$

$$y\text{-direction}: \rho\left(\frac{\partial v}{\partial t} + u\frac{\partial v}{\partial x} + v\frac{\partial v}{\partial y} + w\frac{\partial v}{\partial z}\right) = -\frac{\partial p}{\partial y} + \mu\left(\frac{\partial^2 v}{\partial x^2} + \frac{\partial^2 v}{\partial y^2} + \frac{\partial^2 v}{\partial z^2}\right) \tag{4.2}$$

$$z\text{-direction}: \rho\left(\frac{\partial w}{\partial t} + u\frac{\partial w}{\partial x} + v\frac{\partial w}{\partial y} + w\frac{\partial w}{\partial z}\right) = -\frac{\partial p}{\partial z} + \mu\left(\frac{\partial^2 w}{\partial x^2} + \frac{\partial^2 w}{\partial y^2} + \frac{\partial^2 w}{\partial z^2}\right) \tag{4.3}$$

Equation of continuity is:

$$\frac{\partial \rho}{\partial t} + \frac{\partial(\rho u)}{\partial x} + \frac{\partial(\rho v)}{\partial y} + \frac{\partial(\rho w)}{\partial z} = 0 \tag{4.4}$$

The following assumptions are made here:

(1) Fluid is incompressible.
(2) Order of length along $x$, $y$, $z$ is $x$, $y >> z$.
(3) Order of velocities along $x$, $y$, $z$ are $u$, $v >> w$.
(4) Inertial terms($\rho$) are neglected compared to the pressure and viscosity terms.
(5) Viscosity is brought only by $\partial^2 u/\partial z^2$ and $\partial^2 v/\partial z^2$.

According to the assumptions of (3) and (4), Eq. (4.3) becomes

$$\frac{\partial p}{\partial z} = 0$$

namely the pressure, $p$, becomes uniform along the depth, $z$. According to all the assumptions, Eqs. (4.1) and (4.2) become

$$\frac{\partial p}{\partial x} = \mu \frac{\partial^2 u}{\partial z^2} \tag{4.5}$$

$$\frac{\partial p}{\partial y} = \mu \frac{\partial^2 v}{\partial z^2} \tag{4.6}$$

Boundary conditions are given as follows:

$$u = 0 \text{ at } z = 0, \text{ and } u = U \text{ at } z = h \tag{4.7}$$

When Eqs. (4.5) and (4.6) are integrated along $z$,

$$u = \frac{1}{2\mu}\frac{\partial p}{\partial x}\left(z^2 - hz\right) + \frac{U}{h}(h - z) \tag{4.8}$$

$$v = \frac{1}{2\mu}\frac{\partial p}{\partial y}\left(z^2 - hz\right) \tag{4.9}$$

When we insert these equations into Eq. (4.4), neglecting $w$,

$$\frac{\partial}{\partial x}\left\{\frac{1}{2\mu}\frac{\partial p}{\partial x}\left(z^2 - hz\right) + \frac{U}{h}(h - z)\right\} + \frac{\partial}{\partial y}\left\{\frac{1}{2\mu}\frac{\partial p}{\partial x}\left(z^2 - hz\right)\right\} = 0 \tag{4.10}$$

Integrating the above equation for $0 \le z \le h$, then

$$\frac{\partial}{\partial x}\left\{\frac{1}{2\mu}\frac{\partial p}{\partial x}\left(-\frac{h^3}{6}\right) + \frac{U}{h}\left(\frac{h^2}{2}\right)\right\} + \frac{\partial}{\partial y}\left\{\frac{1}{2\mu}\frac{\partial p}{\partial x}\left(-\frac{h^3}{6}\right)\right\} = 0$$

$$\frac{\partial}{\partial x}\left(h^3\frac{\partial p}{\partial x}\right) + \frac{\partial}{\partial y}\left(h^3\frac{\partial p}{\partial y}\right) = 6\mu U\frac{\partial h}{\partial x} \tag{4.11}$$

This is the two-dimensional Reynolds equation in lubrication. When the geometric depth distribution $h(x, y)$ and the boundary conditions are given, the pressure distribution $p(x, y)$ can be obtained over the gap surface of the bearing.

The expression in polar coordinates is

$$\frac{\partial}{\partial r}\left(h^3 r \frac{\partial p}{\partial r}\right) + \frac{1}{r}\frac{\partial}{\partial \theta}\left(h^3 \frac{\partial p}{\partial \theta}\right) = 6r\omega\mu \frac{\partial h}{\partial \theta} \tag{4.12}$$

where $\omega$ denotes the angular velocity.

When the variation in $y$ direction is ignored for one-dimensional analysis, the Reynolds equation becomes

$$\frac{\partial}{\partial x}\left(h^3 \frac{\partial p}{\partial x}\right) = 6\mu U \frac{\partial h}{\partial x} \tag{4.13}$$

Integrated this equation with respect to $x$, then

$$h^3 \frac{\mathrm{d}p}{\mathrm{d}x} = 6\mu U(h - c) \tag{4.14}$$

where $c$ is an arbitrary constant. When the gap can assume to have a linear slope as $\frac{\mathrm{d}h}{\mathrm{d}x} = \frac{h_2 - h_1}{L}$ where $L$ denotes the length of gap and $(\ )_1$ inlet and $(\ )_2$ outlet,

$$\frac{\mathrm{d}p}{\mathrm{d}h} = \frac{\mathrm{d}p}{\mathrm{d}x}\frac{\mathrm{d}x}{\mathrm{d}h} = 6\mu U \frac{h - h_0}{h^3}\frac{L}{h_2 - h_1}$$

When the above equation is integrated, assuming the pressure $p = 0$ at $h_1$ and $h_2$, then

$$p(h) = \frac{6\mu UL}{h^2}\frac{(h_1 - h)(h - h_2)}{{h_1}^2 - {h_2}^2} \tag{4.15}$$

This implies that the pressure $p > 0$ if $h_1 > h > h_2$ and that the pressure $p$ is proportional to the velocity $U$ and the length $L$ and inversely proportional to $h^2$.

Or Eq. (4.14) is rewritten as

$$\frac{\mathrm{d}p}{\mathrm{d}x} = 6\mu U\left(\frac{1}{h^2} - \frac{c}{h^3}\right); \quad h = h(x)$$

and is directly integrated with respect to $x$, then

$$p(x) = p_0 + 6\mu U \int \left(\frac{1}{h^2} - \frac{c}{h^3}\right) dx; \quad p = p_0 \ at \ x = 0 \ and \ L \tag{4.16}$$

# References

1. Yamane, T., Maruyama, O., Nishida, M., Kosaka, R.: Research and development of a monopivot centrifugal blood pump for clinical use: collaboration for a product between medical and engineering teams. Adv. Indust. Sci. Technol. **5**(1), 17–24 (2012), Synthesiology English edition
2. Hoshi, H., Shinshi, T., Takatani, S.: Third-generation blood pumps with mechanical noncontact magnetic bearing. J. Artif. Organs **30**(5), 324–338 (2006). Blackwell
3. Maruyama, O., Nishida, M., Tsutsui, T., Jikuya, T., Yamane, T.: The hemolytic characteristics of monopivot magnetic suspension blood pumps with washout holes. J. Artif. Organs **29**(4), 345–348 (2005). Blackwell
4. Tagi, A., Miyazaki, M., Mochiwaki, A., Yamane, T.: Study on hemolysis reduction due to bearing friction of a centrifugal blood pump. In: Proceedings of frontier conference, The Society of Life Support Engineering, March 2015 (in Japanese)
5. Kosaka, R., Maruyama, O., Nishida, M., Yada, T., Saito, S., Hirai, S., Yamane, T.: Improvement of hemocompatibility in centrifugal blood pump with hydrodynamic bearings and semi-open impeller: in vitro evaluation. J. Artif. Organs **33**(10), 798–804 (2009). Wiley-Blackwell
6. Hori, Y.: Hydrodynamic Lubrication. Springer, New York (2006)

# Chapter 5
# Motor, Battery, and Magnetic Suspension

## 5.1 Motor Mechanism

A driving motor is also an important component. Brushless DC motors are most frequently applied to VADs. In the brushless DC motor, the stator is composed of coils rotating a magnetic field and the rotor is composed of permanent magnets. The way of switching current to form a rotating pair of poles is shown in Fig. 5.1. It can be recognized that only a pair of coils is activated simultaneously. To prevent cogging, namely fluctuation of rotational speed, the numbers of rotor/stator poles are selected to be different such as 6-poles for a stator and 8-poles for a rotor.

## 5.2 Battery and Cable

Most of VADs have a power source composed of lithium-ion or nickel-cadmium battery. A patient often carries two batteries when he/she goes out and simultaneously two batteries are being charged at home.

Cables are designed as soft as possible to be easily bent but as strong as possible not to be broken by fatigue. Since cable infection is a severe clinical problem, the cable should not have gaps between skins at the penetration port.

Therefore a wireless transcutaneous energy transmission system, TETS, is requested from clinical side. However, it is not so easy to keep sufficient reliability and anatomical fit compared with a wired system. Sooner or later VADs with TETS would be provided by some manufacturers.



T. Yamane, *Mechanism of Artificial Heart*, DOI 10.1007/978-4-431-55831-6_5

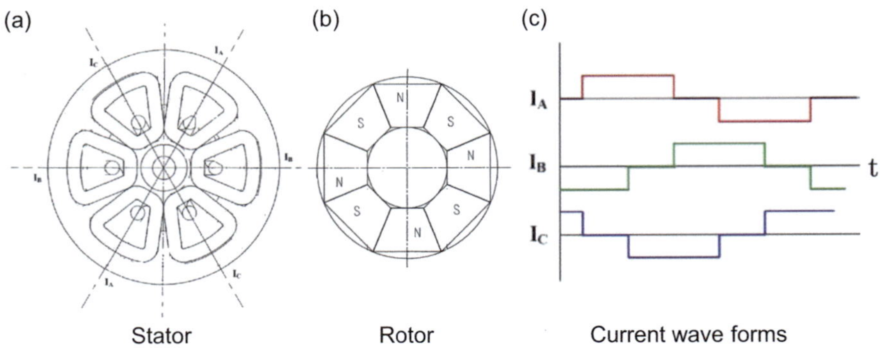


**Fig. 5.1** Mechanism of a brushless DC motor (Reproduced with partial modification and with permission of Citizen Chiba Precision Co., Ltd.)

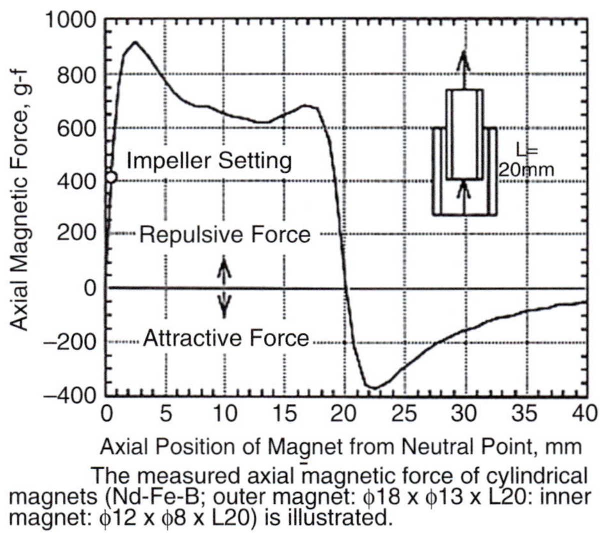


**Fig. 5.2** Axial force characteristics of permanent magnet rings [1]

## 5.3 Magnetic Suspension

When we use permanent magnet for magnetic coupling or for magnetic suspension, we should understand an important theorem. Anything cannot be supported only by permanent magnets freely in a three-dimensional space without any stabilization control or without super conductivity. This is called as Earnshaw's theorem in magnetic fields. When we use rare-earth permanent magnets such as Nd-Fe-B, Sm-Co, we should be careful to their strong magnetic force. We should understand not only the radial repulsive force but also special axial force behavior such as shown in Fig. 5.2.

## Reference

1. Yamane, T., Ikeda, T., Orita, T., Tsuitsui, T., Jikuya, T.: Design of a centrifugal blood pump with magnetic suspension. Artif Organs **19**(7), 625–630 (1995)

# Chapter 6
# Flow Visualization and Computational Fluid Dynamic Analysis

## 6.1 Particle Image Velocimetry (PIV)

Flow visualization reveals the environments where blood is exposed. Though the tracer particles do not indicate the behavior of blood cells, they show flow velocity correctly when the size is as small as to trace the streamlines.

Apparatus (Fig. 6.1): The pump model is filled with 64 % NaI water solution with a matched refractive index to acrylic resin (being 1.49). The images of $SiO_2$ beads (0.15-mm sphere), having the same density as the liquid ($1.9 \times 10^3$ kg/m$^3$), are suspended in the circuit. One of the imaging methods is to use double-pulse YAG laser with a short interval such as 1 μs interval and to transfer the two images to continuous two frames of regular video camera (with 1/30 s frame interval).

Another imaging method, for a particle tracking method, is to use a high-speed video camera (e.g., a frame rate of 4500 frame/s), and the particles are illuminated by a continuous laser light sheet (e.g., 4 – W Ar – ion laser).

### 6.1.1 *Visualization of a Centrifugal Blood Pump*

Similarity law: A 300 % scale-up visualization model is made with acrylic resin and is based on Reynolds similarity law, especially regarding the blood contacting geometry. The surface of the model is polished to the roughness of Ra $<$ 0.2 μm. The experimental conditions should be set based on the strict Reynolds similarity law, namely a 1/15 rotational speed and a $1.8 \times$ flow rate.

Particle image analysis (Fig. 6.2): A method of analysis is a particle tracking velocimetry (PTV). (a) The four-frame tracking method can be used for in-plane motion to eliminate inaccurate particle images that cannot be traced for continuous four frames. A PTV has a fine spatial resolution even near the surface wall. (b) The three-frame tracking method or the spring-model tracking method can be used to



T. Yamane, *Mechanism of Artificial Heart*, DOI 10.1007/978-4-431-55831-6_6

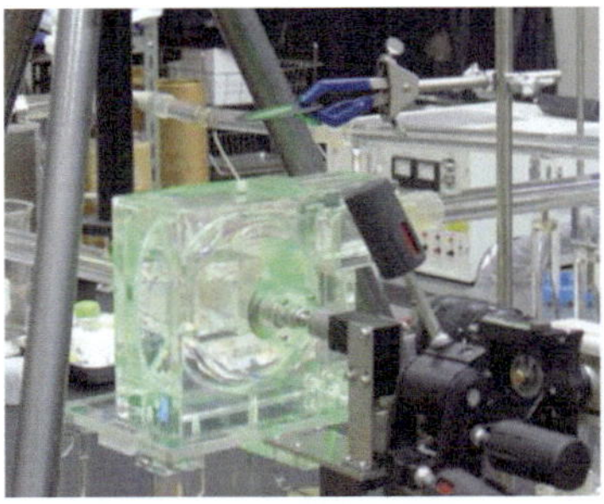

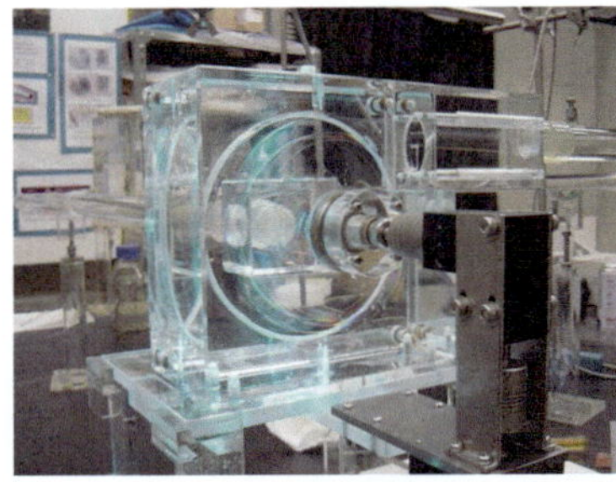

| | | |
|---|---|---|
| Apparatus | Acrylic 2.5x model | |
| | Video camera (30frame/s) | |
| | Double pulse YAG laser sheet (500μs) | |
| Fluid | 64wt%NaI aq (refluctive index: 1.49, specific gravity: 1.9) | |
| Tracer | Silver coated glass beads (ϕ10 μm) | |
| Analysis | Cross-correlation method | |

| | |
|---|---|
| Apparatus | Acrylic 2.5x model |
| | High-speed Video camera (4500f/s, ring) |
| | Ar-ion laser light sheet (3-4W) |
| Fluid | 64wt%NaI aq (refluctive index: 1.49, specific gravity: 1.9) |
| Tracer | $SiO_2$ beads (ϕ150 μm) |
| Analysis | 4-frame particle tracking method |

**Fig. 6.1** Experimental apparatus for flow visualization, (**a**) with a double-pulse laser (**b**) with a continuous laser

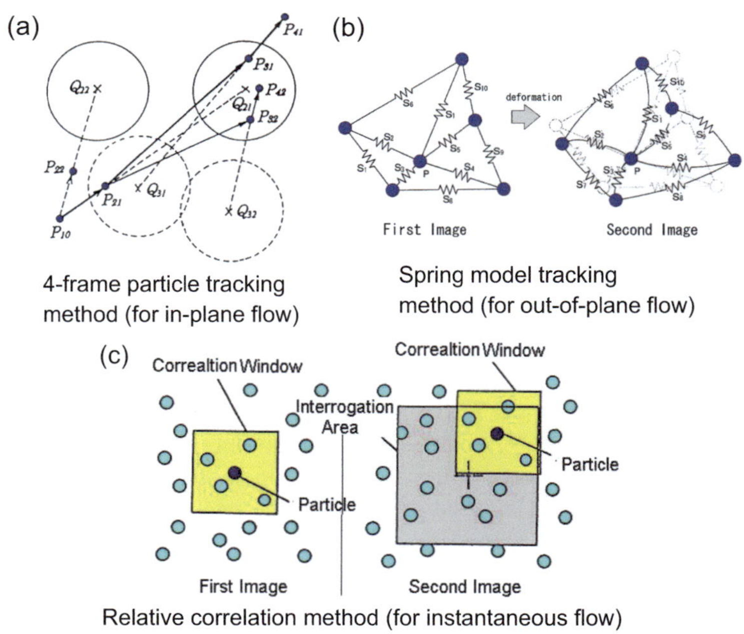


**Fig. 6.2** Analyses for particle image velocimetry (PIV)

evaluate the secondary flow of out-of-plane motion since particle images are captured only for two or three frames during penetration of the laser light sheet, whose thickness is 1.6 mm.

(c) The other is a particle image correlation velocimetry (called PICV here), which finds the highest correlation points for several particles and derives a vector averaging several particles. Regarding the necessary resolution, the resolution was tuned up to obtain the sufficient contours of shear rate as shown in Results.

Sample results are shown here for a centrifugal pump. In the planar view from the tip of vanes to a volute, a flow from a vane is visualized to land smoothly on the surface of a casing or a volute (Fig. 6.3). In the vertical view from the tip of vanes to a volute, a formation of a jet from a vane is well visualized.

At the bifurcation point to the outlet, so-called a tongue, flow separation should be avoided. In a case of a separation, standing vortex is observed at the tongue region in flow visualization, shown in left part of Fig. 6.4; correspondingly a thrombus is formed along volute surface from the tongue in an animal test. It can be removed by a design of round tongue, as shown in right part of Fig. 6.4, then thrombus formation was avoided in an animal test. It indicates that flow visualization can estimate thrombus formation point but cannot estimate thrombus growth.

Flow visualization was conducted for 300 % scale-up model of the SunMedical centrifugal VAD (Fig. 6.5). The flow visualization revealed a sufficient blood wash between rotating vanes and a stationary shaft.

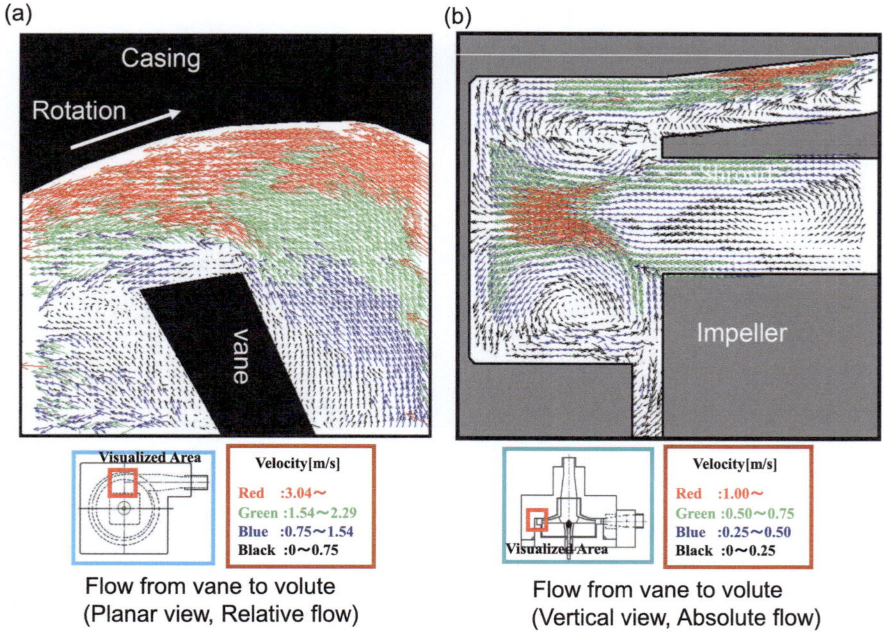


**Fig. 6.3** A flow visualization result for impeller tip region [1]

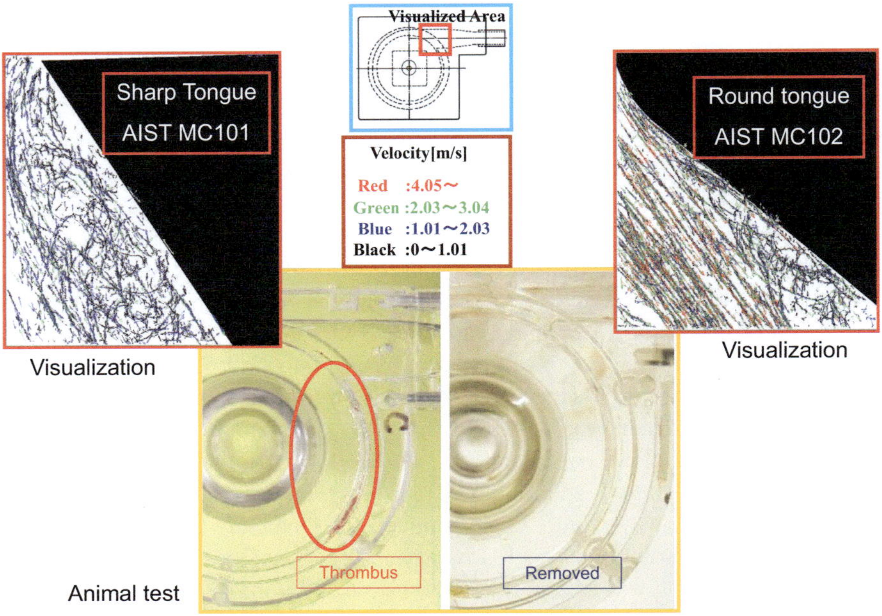


**Fig. 6.4** A flow visualization result for tongue regions [1]

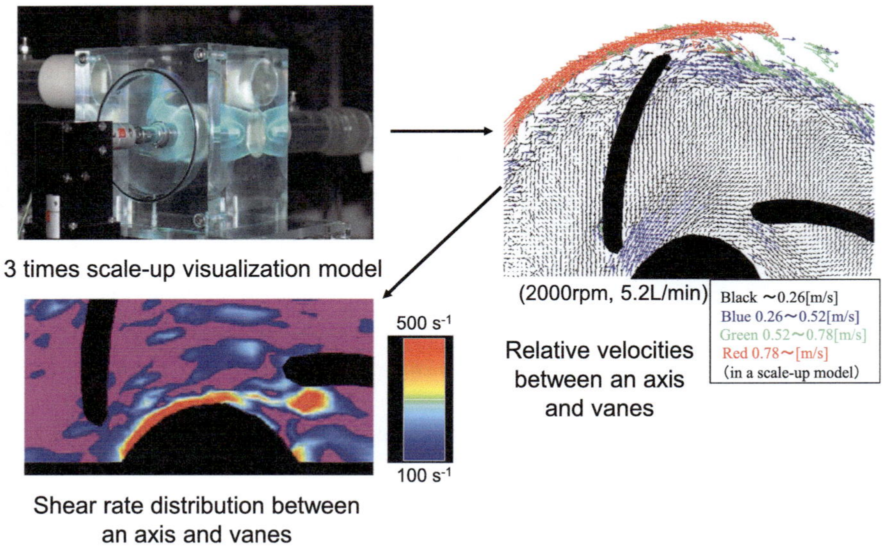


**Fig. 6.5** Flow visualization for EVAHEART [2] (Reproduced with permission of Sun Medical Technology Research Corp. and Tokyo Women's Medical University)

### *6.1.2 Visualization Regarding Washout Hole Flow*

Around a pivot bearing, blood wash is necessary. Though the tangential flow is accelerated to the tip of impeller and most of them go to the outlet, some of them returns to inlet direction through the top gap or the bottom gap, keeping its angular momentum, namely (velocity x radius), constant. If we see the flow from the side carefully, radially returning flow to the center, so-called secondary flow, may be seen through precise flow visualization analysis. Figure 6.6 shows that the secondary flow does not reach the pivot at the center for washout holes whose diameter is 9 mm and 8 mm, but it reaches the pivot for those with 7 mm and 6 mm diameter. It was found that the blood wash improves when the washout hole diameter is less than 7 mm.

Second interesting result of flow visualization regarding washout flow is a relative tangential velocity through the top gap or the bottom gap of the impeller. As I wrote, the flow at the impeller tip returns to the center keeping the momentum, namely increasing the tangential velocity. Then the tangential flow reaches the impeller rotational velocity, and the relative velocity between the impeller and the blood becomes zero at a certain radius.

Figure 6.7 shows the radial distribution of the tangential velocity of the blood and of the impeller. Figure 6.7 is a picture of canine experiment of an extracorporeal centrifugal pump, whose impeller is semi-open type. White circle was able to be seen after the experiment and that is presumably a platelet deposition, which is not harmful to human operation.

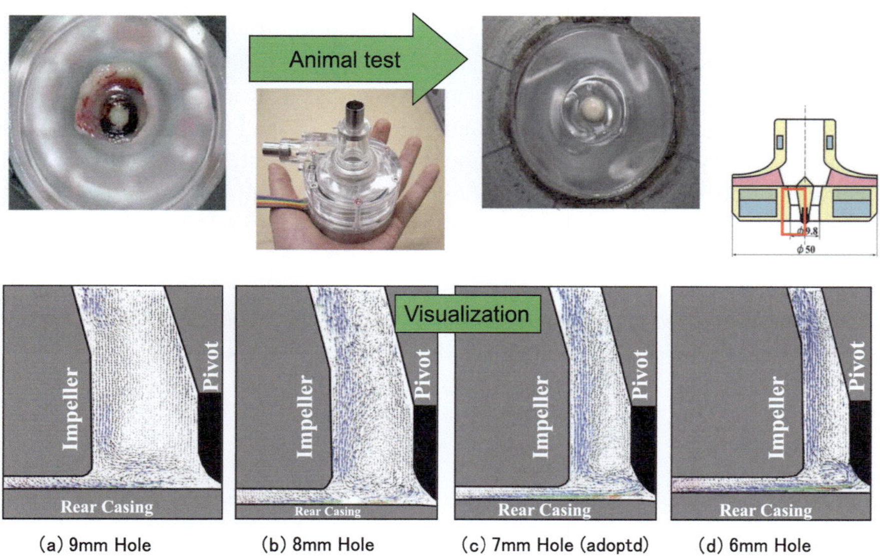


**Fig. 6.6** Visualization results for washout hole regions [3]

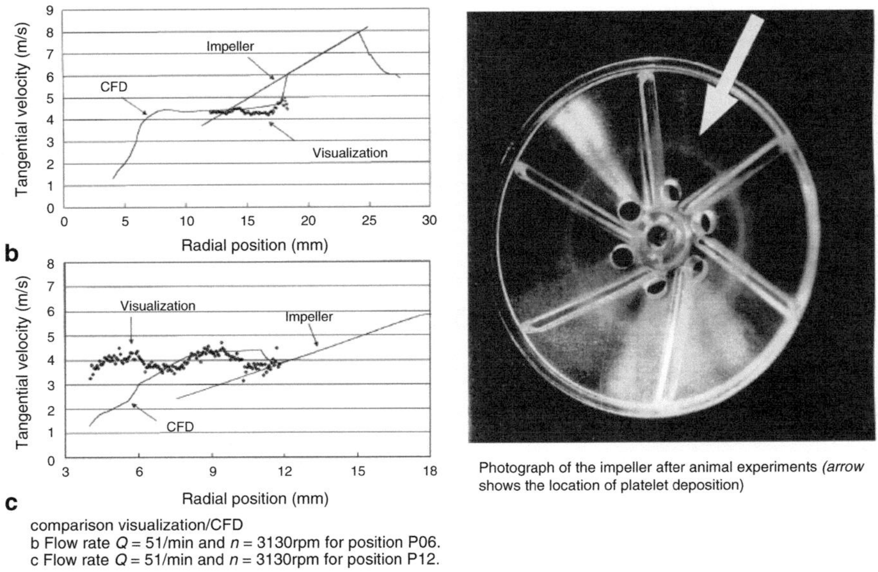


**Fig. 6.7** Comparison of a circular region of platelet deposition observed in an animal test and a region of zero relative velocity observed in a flow visualization [4]

## *6.1.3 Visualization of a Gap Flow in a Centrifugal Blood Pump*

One of the interesting applications of flow visualization is a gap flow in a centrifugal blood pump. The flow channels, in general, are composed of narrow gaps in a centrifugal pump. Gap flow between a rotating disk and a stationary wall was studied by Daily and Nece [5], Ketola and McGrew [6], and Cooper and Reshotko [7]. There are two Reynolds numbers governing the flow patterns, namely the radial Reynolds number, $\omega R^2/\nu$, and the gap Reynolds number, $s\omega R/\nu$, where $R$ denotes an impeller radius, $s$ a gap width, $\omega$ a rotational speed, and $\nu$ a kinematic viscosity. When the gap Reynolds number is replaced by a spacing ratio, $s/R$, the gap flow profiles can be classified empirically in four regimes as Fig. 6.8. Regime I and II correspond to merged and separate laminar boundary layers, and Regime III and IV correspond to merged and separate turbulent boundary layers, respectively.

Our experiments with flow visualization were as follows.

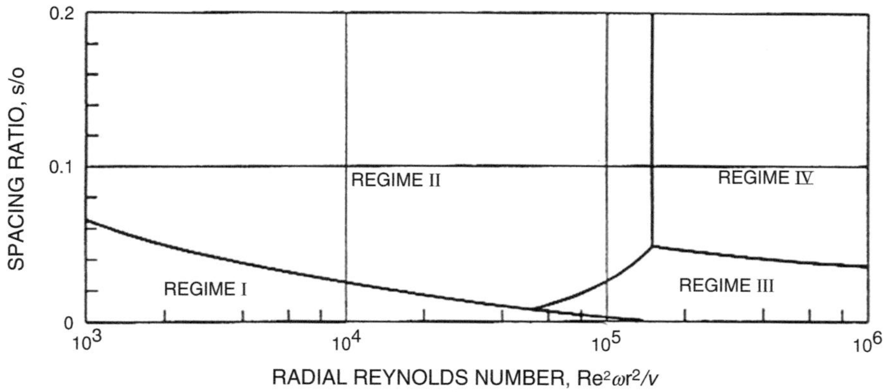


**Fig. 6.8** Gap flow characteristics in a centrifugal blood pump [6] (Regime I: Laminar flow, merged boundary layers; Regime II: Laminar flow, separate boundary layers; Regime III: Turbulent flow, merged boundary layers; Regime IV: Turbulent flow, separate boundary layers)

**Gap Flow Velocity Profiles**

The tangential velocity, $u$, was normalized with the impeller tip speed, $U_2$. The distance from the casing, $z$, was normalized with the gap width, $s$. The gap flow profiles were viewed as scatter graphs (Fig. 6.9). By the least squared method, a curve was fitted consisting of a constant velocity core region and two parabolic boundary layers of width δa, casing side, and δb, impeller side. This is a suitable approximation for Reynolds numbers within the range $10^4 < Re < 10^5$.

**Effect of Specific Speed**

The specific speed, representing root of a ratio of circumferential velocity to radial velocity, is governed mainly by the external resistance. The radial Reynolds number was kept constant as $Re = 5.9 \times 10^4$ during the experiment (Fig. 6.10). As the specific speed increases, there is little change in the gap tangential velocity profile as long as $Re$ is kept constant. The total extent of the boundary layers is approximately 50 % of the gap width.

**Effect of Reynolds Number**

The radial Reynolds number, $Re = \mathrm{R}^2\omega/v$, is governed mainly by the rotational speed, $\omega$. The specific speed is kept constant as $n_s = 158$ during the experiment. The extent of the core region increases with increasing $Re$, and the velocity of the core region decreases. At higher $Re$ the widths of the boundary layers are smaller. The impeller side boundary layer is always narrower than that at the casing side. The total thickness of the boundary layer varies from 30 to 60 % of the gap width.

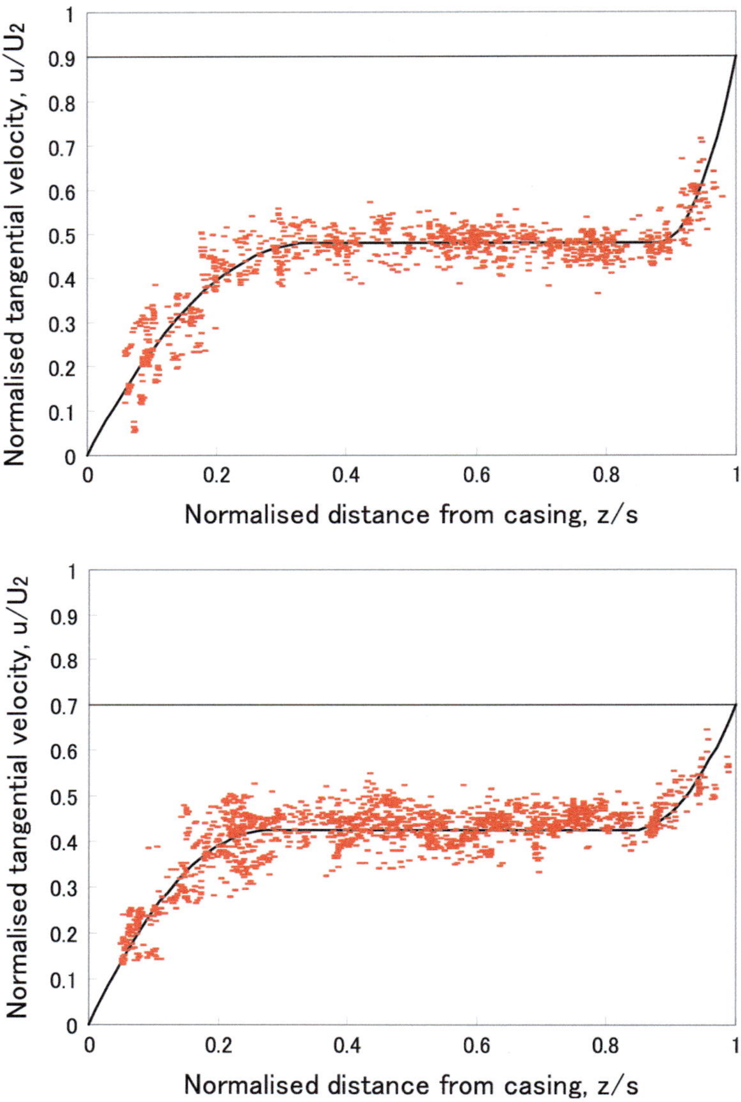


**Fig. 6.9** Gap flow profiles in a centrifugal blood pump [8]

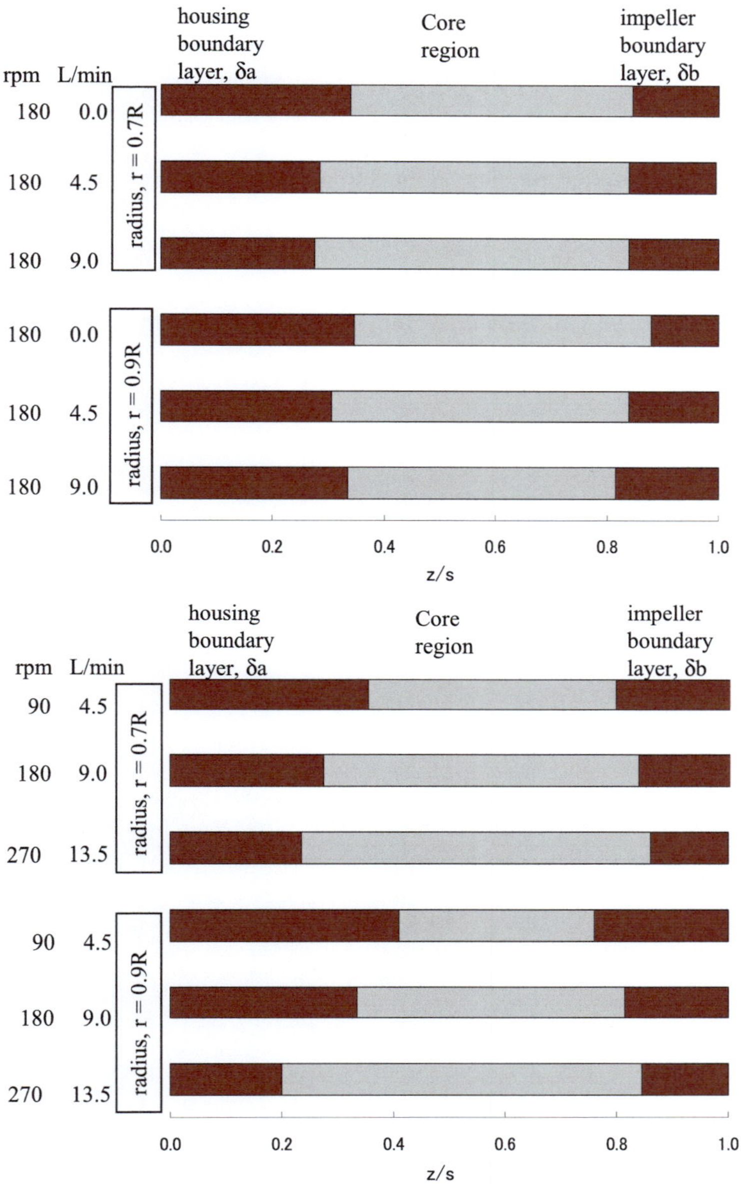


**Fig. 6.10** Effects of specific speed and Reynolds number to velocity profiles [8]

## 6.2 Computational Fluid Dynamic (CFD) Analysis

The purpose of a computational fluid dynamic (CFD) analysis is to assess hydraulic performance, risk of hemolysis/thrombus formation, or risk of cavitation, in ISO 14708-5, [9].

(a) Device hydraulic performance: A device design can be evaluated in producing specified hydraulic output within acceptable efficiency.
(b) Risk of hemolysis or thrombus formation: Shear stress, exposure time, and their history for blood cells inside the device that could cause blood trauma can be evaluated. Separation and stagnation zones are to be analyzed associated with a risk of thrombus formation.
(c) Risk of cavitation: The risk of air emboli, blood cell damage, and blood contacting surfaces damage associated with possible low-pressure zones inside the device can be evaluated.

However, the use is limited to the design stage and to the relative value evaluation since the absolute values need careful validation.

The following items govern the results of CFD analyses:

1. Mesh/grid generation such as mesh size
2. Used mathematical model such as k-ε turbulence model or laminar flow model
3. Boundary conditions and initial conditions

Separate evaluation should be conducted with regard to the following items:

1. Validation (code verification and solution verification)
2. Error analysis (uncertainty quantification)
3. Sensitivity analysis with respect to input parameters

Since the CFD analysis often fails in obtaining correct pressures or stresses, pressure-related evaluation such as pump pressure validation needs to be conducted.

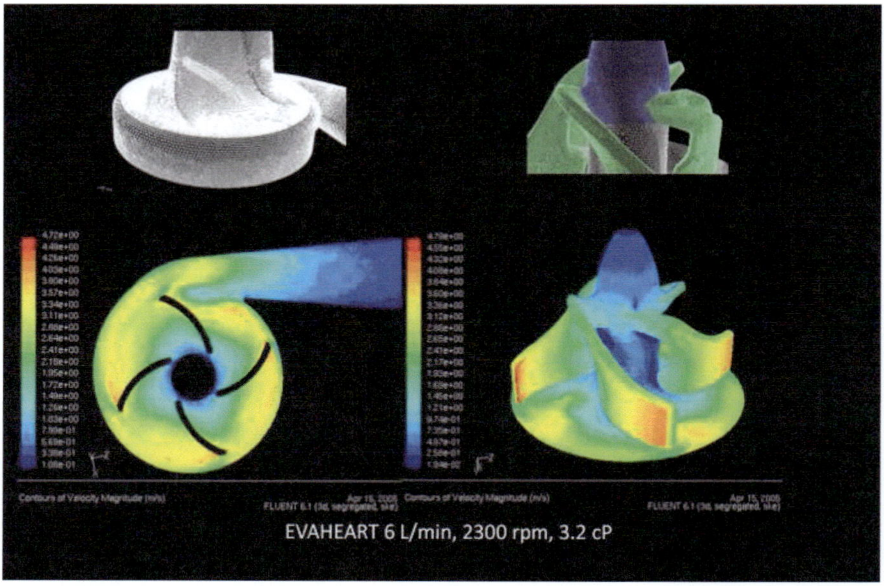


**Fig. 6.11** Velocity profile based on computational fluid dynamic (CFD) analysis for EVAHEART (Reproduced with permission of Sun Medical Technology Research Corp. and Tokyo Women's Medical University)

Figure 6.11 represents a CFD analysis for a velocity profile of the EVAHEART ventricular assist system.

## 6.3 Similarity Laws: Development Tool

### 6.3.1 *Similarity Law 1:* Reynolds Number

One of the fluid dynamic similarity conditions for geometrically similar models is coincidence of Reynolds numbers and ratio of inertial and viscous forces. This leads to similarity of "velocity size." The 2D equation of motion for viscous fluid without external forces is as follows:

$$\frac{\mathrm{D}u}{\mathrm{D}t} = -\frac{1}{\rho}\frac{\partial p}{\partial \mathrm{x}} + \frac{\mu}{\rho}\left(\frac{\partial^2 u}{\partial x^2} + \frac{\partial^2 u}{\partial y^2}\right); \quad \frac{\mathrm{D}}{\mathrm{D}t} \equiv \frac{\partial}{\partial t} + u\frac{\partial}{\partial x} + v\frac{\partial}{\partial y}$$

Dimensional analysis is conducted here to find similarity law. When the position *x, y, z* are divided by typical length *L*, velocity *u, v, w* by typical velocity *U*, and time *t* by *L*/*U*, and *p*/*r by* $U^2$, then the non-dimensional values are denoted by $(\,)'$, then the above equation becomes

$$\frac{U^2}{L}\frac{\mathrm{D}u'}{\mathrm{D}t'} = -\frac{U^2}{L}\frac{\partial p'}{\partial \mathrm{x}'} + \frac{\mu U}{\rho L^2}\nabla^2 u' \qquad \frac{\mathrm{D}u'}{\mathrm{D}t'} = -\frac{\partial p'}{\partial \mathrm{x}'} + \frac{\mu}{\rho U L}\nabla^2 u'$$

Therefore, to achieve a fluid dynamic similarity for different sizes or different densities or viscosities, a parameter

$$\mathrm{Re} = \frac{\rho U L}{\mu}$$

should be coincided. The result is the same as in *y* direction. This is called the Reynolds similarity law and the parameter *Re* is called "Reynolds number."

### 6.3.2 *Similarity Law 2:* Specific Speed

The second similarity law for rotary fluid machine is related to the coincidence of "velocity orientation," representing the ratio of fluid velocity $U_a$ consisting the outlet flow rate and rotating velocity of an impeller $U_r$. It should satisfy, with flow rate *Q*, impeller rotational speed *ω*, and typical length *L*, the following equation:

$$U_a/U_r = \left(Q/L^2\right)/(\omega L) = \text{const. namely } Q/\omega L^3 = \text{const.} \tag{6.1}$$

When the typical length $L$, such as impeller radius, is replaced by a theoretical pump head $H$ and rotational speed $\omega$,

$$gH = p/\rho = \eta(\omega L)^2$$

Then

$$H/(\omega L)^2 = \eta/g \tag{6.2}$$

where the right hand side is almost a constant.

$$1/L^3 = \omega^3 H^{-3/2}(\eta/g)^{3/2}$$

can be substituted into Eq. (6.1), a similarity condition

$$\omega^2 Q H^{-3/2} = \text{const.}$$

can be derived and the square root of the above is

$$n_S \equiv \omega Q^{1/2} H^{-3/4} = \text{const.}$$

Where $n_s$ is called a specific speed and has unit of (rpm)(L/min)$^{1/2}$(m)$^{-3/4}$. The specific speed is obtained by taking the square root of Eq. (6.1), then the specific speed represents

$$n_S \propto \sqrt{U_a/U_r}$$

Alternatively when the Eq. (6.1) is satisfied, the velocity orientation becomes similar.

On the other hand, since the highest efficiency for each pump is achieved at a certain special specific speed, the specific speed can be used by industries to select a suitable pump type among variety of pump types.

### *6.3.3 Meaning of the Variation of the Two Similarity Parameters for a Pump*

The two similarity parameters can be used not only for similar experiments but also for operational conditions of a single pump.

1. Constant Reynolds number conditions correspond approximately to constant rotational speed conditions.
2. Constant specific speed conditions correspond to constant outlet velocity/rotational velocity ratios, $U_a/U_r = Q/\omega L^3$, which can be approximately attained with constant resistance.

The two curves are almost orthogonal on a pressure-flow plane (P – Q).

## References


1. Yamane, T., Maruyama, O., Nishida, M., Kosaka, R., Chida, T., Kawamura, H., Kuwana, K., Ishihara, K., Sankai, Y., Matsuzaki, M., Shigeta, O., Enomoto, Y., Tsutsui, T.: Antithrombogenic properties of a monopivot magnetic-suspension centrifugal pump for circulatory assist. J. Artif. Organs **32**(6), 484–489 (2008). Wiley-Blackwell
2. Yamane, T., Nishida, M., Kawamura, H., Miyakoshi, T., Yamazaki, K.: Flow visualization for the implantable ventricular assist device EVAHEART®. J. Artif. Organs **16**, 42–48 (2013). Springer
3. Yamane, T., Maruyama, O., Nishida, M., Toyoda, M., Tsutsui, T., Jikuya, T., Shigeta, O., Sankai, Y.: The Most profitable use of flow visualization in the elimination of thrombus from a monopivot magnetic suspension blood pump. J. Artif. Organs **28**(4), 390–397 (2004). Blackwell
4. Aouidef, A., Yamane, T., Nishida, M., Toyoda, M., Tsukamoto, Y., Konishi, Y., Masuzawa, T., Tsukiya, T., Taenaka, Y.: Flow visualization analysis of relative stagnation areas on the impeller surface of a centrifugal blood pump. J. Artif. Organs **4**(4), 262–268 (2001). JSAO
5. Daily, J.W., Nece, R.E.: Chamber dimension effects on induced flow and frictional resistance of enclosed rotating disks. J. Basic Eng., Trans. ASME **59**(9), 218–229 (1960)
6. Ketola, H.N., McGrew, J.M.: Pressure, frictional resistance, and flow characteristics of the partially wetted rotating disk. J. Lubr. Technol., Trans. ASME **90**, 395–404 (1968)
7. Cooper, P., Reshotko, E.: Turbulent flow between a rotating disk and a parallel wall. AIAA J. **13** (5), 573–578 (1975)
8. Yamanae, T., Clarke, H., Asztalos, B., Nishida, M., Kobayashi, T.: Flow visualization measurement for shear velocity distribution in the impeller-casing gap of a centrifugal blood pump. JSME Int. J. Ser. C **42**(3), 621–627 (1999)
9. ISO 14708-5, Implants for surgery — Active implantable medical devices — Part 5: Circulatory support devices (2010)

# Chapter 7
# How Do We Select Materials?

## 7.1 Pump Material

Pump materials have been selected based on both hemocompatibility and structural strength.

For pulsatile TAHs/VADs, polyurethane is often used as pump material because of possessing both hemocompatibility and structural strength. Polytetrafluoroethylene (PTFE) is also used for endovascular grafts.

For extracorporeal rotary pumps, polycarbonate is often used as short-term hemocompatible/structural material because of the toughness against impact and the transparency for observation of blood.

At present for almost all implantable rotary VADs, titanium or titanium alloy as Ti-6Al-4V polished to submicron surface roughness, are used as pump material because other metals have been reported a certain lack of biocompatibility.

Not much new materials have been introduced since getting approval to a new material needs clinical evidences.

## 7.2 Coating Material

Typical hemocompatible coating material is heparin and 2-methacryloyloxyethyl phosphorylcholine (MPC) polymer. Diamond-like carbon (DLC) can also be coated on hard materials. Heparin coating is used for DuraHeart and MPC polymer coating is used for EVAHEART. On the other hand, Avcothane was coated on segmented polyurethane for pulsatile VADs.



T. Yamane, *Mechanism of Artificial Heart*, DOI 10.1007/978-4-431-55831-6_7

## 7.3 Bearing Material

A comparative study for materials against rotational wear will be explained here.

To compare the bearing materials, a pivot bearing was modeled as a ball and a plate, and the rotating wear tests were conducted with a rotating wear machine. The ball was attached to a rotating shaft through a Teflon socket, and a cubic receptor was inserted into a stationary square pit in a vessel and axially loaded. They were dipped in a small saline vessel whose temperature was kept at 37′C. To prevent splash several fins and a cover plate were provided to the vessel. The rotational speed of a ball was kept at 2000 rpm and the axial load to a receptor was kept at 1 kg or 2 kg. The dried weights of balls/sockets and receptors were measured before a test using a precise balance whose accuracy was +1 μg. Each rotational wear test was conducted for 16 h. After the test, the dry weights of the components were measured again and the weight losses were evaluated.

Four kinds of ceramics ($S_{i3}N_4$, $S_iC$, $Al_2O_3$, and $Z_rO_2$) in diameter of 1.59, 3.18, and 3.97 mm were used for pivot balls. Two kinds of materials ($Si_3N_4$ and Ultra high molecular weight polyethylene (UHMWPE )) were used for pivot receptors whose size were 6 × 6 × 4.9 mm.

First wear vs. time was measured by stopping the apparatus at each sampling time (Fig. 7.1). It was found that the loss of weight was almost linear with respect to time.

Then eight kinds of material combinations were tested using ceramic balls of 3.97 mm (Fig. 7.2). It was found that the UHMWPE receptor can reduce the wear amount by 70–90 % compared to the $Si_3N_4$ receptor for different ball diameters. The effects of the ball diameter and the axial load were also compared for a combination of $Si_3N_4$/UHMWPE (Fig. 7.3). The minimum wear amount was found for a combination of a ball diameter of 3 mm though the difference was not so clear for axial loads of 1 kg or 2 kg. A microscopic observation found that coaxial scratch marks were found for a combination of Al2O3/Si3N4 but that the

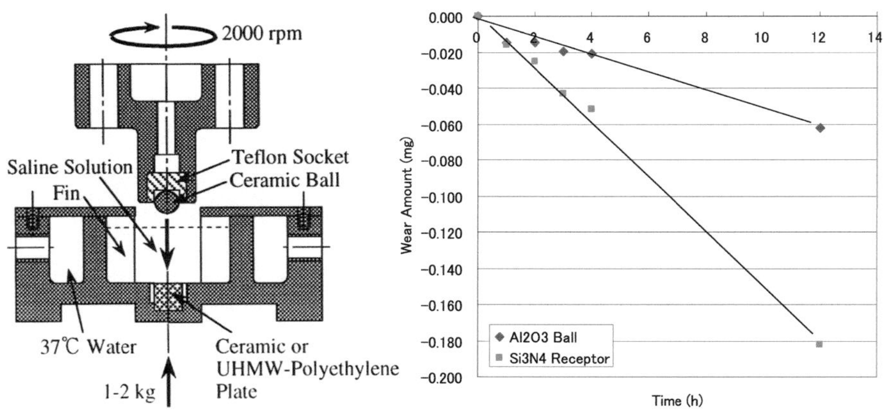


**Fig. 7.1** Time history for rotating wear of pivot materials [1]

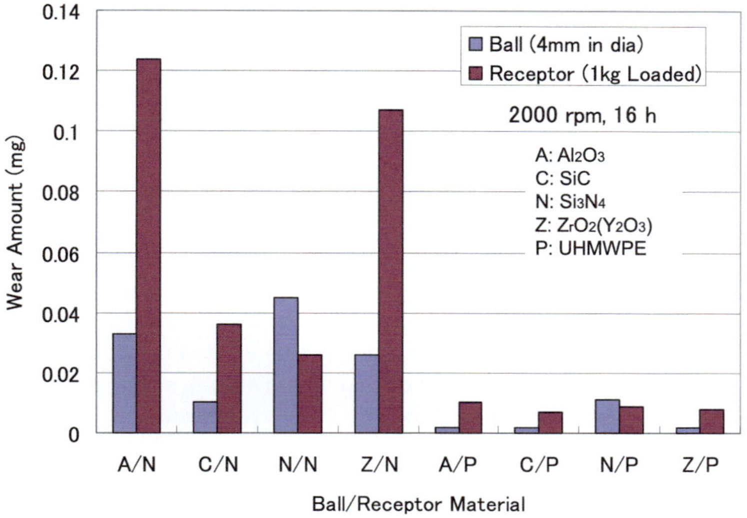


**Fig. 7.2** Comparison of rotating wear for pivot materials [1]

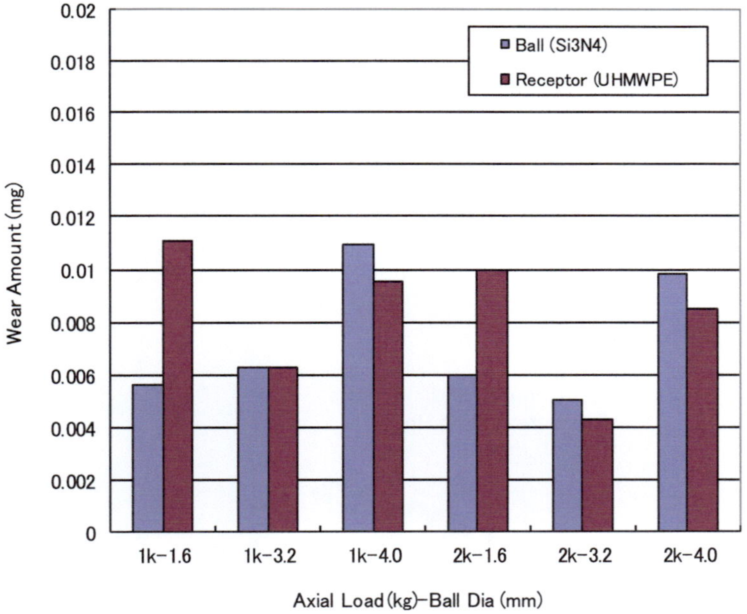


**Fig. 7.3** Comparison of rotating wear for pivot materials [1]

surface of a ball was so smooth for a combination of $Al_2O_3$/UHMWPE. A calculated Hertz pressure, on $Al_2O_3$ ball of around 3 mm in diameter, showed a large difference, namely 1890 MPa for $Si_3M_4$ receptor and 45 MPa for UHMWPE receptor.

This study revealed that the minimum wear for a bearing of a blood pump was attained with a combination of a ceramic ball and an UHMWPE receptor. This happens to coincide with a case of hip joint.

## 7.4 Durability Testing

To evaluate system reliability, a closed circuit is filled with a suitable liquid at 37°C and the test was continued for a target duration. The testing concept and method are described in ISO 14708-5 [4]. System reliability is defined as the probability of a system to perform its function for a specified period of time under stated conditions (for example, the demonstrated reliability of the VAD system shall be X with at least Y confidence for a Z year mission life). The number of systems to be tested under controlled in vitro conditions shall be statistically justified to demonstrate that the stated reliability specifications are met. Statistical methods to be employed in the analysis of the reliability test results shall be described. An example of such a statistical justification is a Weibull calculation.

Japanese guidance for ventricular assist devices/total artificial hearts, which is compatible to ISO 14708-5, is also applicable to Japanese application for approval.

All implanted components shall be tested in a simulated physiological environment, such as a pH buffered, temperature controlled, saline filled tank, and operated within a pulsatile mock circulatory loop. If a pulsatile mock loop is not to be used, a scientific justification shall be provided that lack of pulsatility will not invalidate the test.

For example, a monopivot centrifugal pump, pivot wear was measured continuously for 4 weeks as the distance between the upper casing and the upper impeller surface, using a laser focus displacement meter (Fig. 7.4).

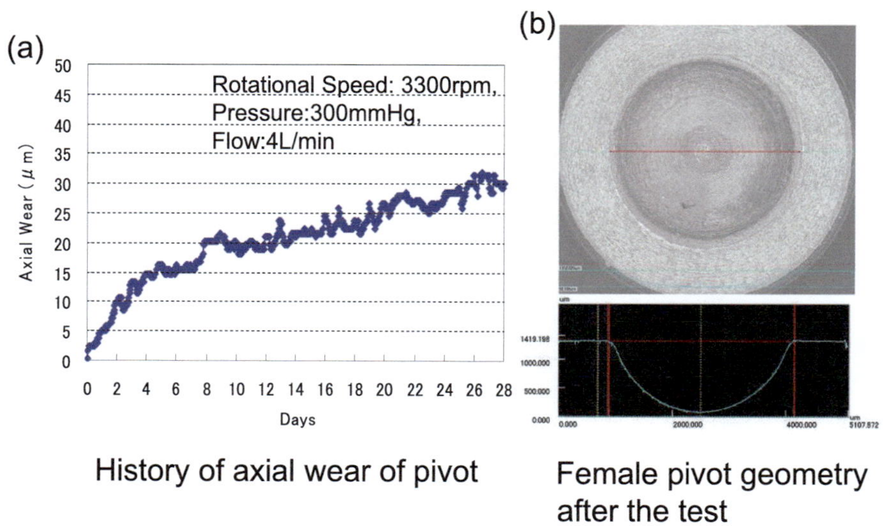


Fig. 7.4 Durability testing for a surgical centrifugal pump [2]

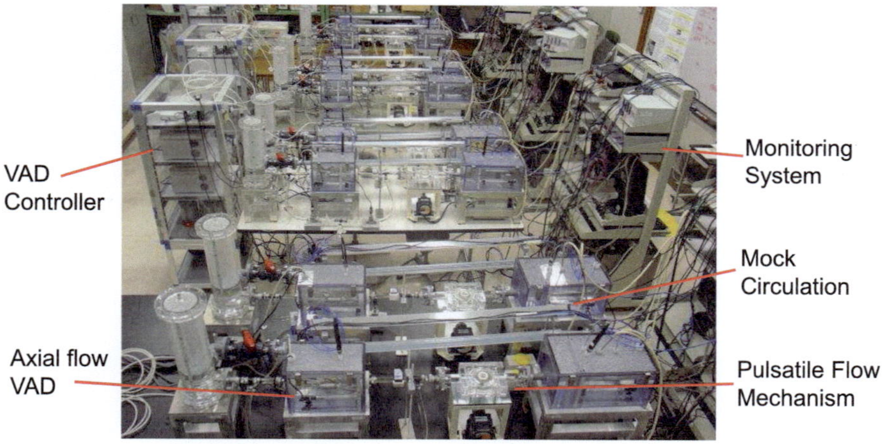


**Fig. 7.5** Durability testing with a pulsatile flow for an axial flow VAD, 8 systems for 2 years [3] (Reproduced with permission of NEDO and AIST)

Another example is a durability testing with pulsatile flow of 0–10 L/min was conducted for 2 years with eight axial flow pumps developed in a NEDO project (Fig. 7.5).

## References

1. Yamane, T., Maruyama, O., Mizuhara, K., Nishida, M., Nonaka, K., Tateishi, T.: Durability enhancement of monopivot magnetic suspension blood pump. J. Congest. Heart Fail. Circ. Support **1**(4), 317–320 (2001)
2. Yamane, T., Kosaka, R., Nishida, M., Maruyama, O., Yamamoto, Y., Kuwana, K., Kawamura, H., Shiraishi, Y., Yambe, T., Sankai, Y., Tsutsui, T.: Hemocompatibility of the MERA Monopivot Centrifugal Pump: toward medium-term use. J. Artif. Organs **37**(2), 217–225 (2013). Wiley-Blackwell
3. Nishida, M., Kosaksa, R., Maruyama, O., Yamane, T., Okubo, T., Hoshi, H., Osada, T., Shirasu, A, Tatsumi, E., Taenaka, Y.: Durability test of the continuous flow ventricular assist devices under pulsatile flow. In: Proceedings of 2011 congress of the Japanese Society for Rotary Blood Pumps, November, p. 23 (2011) (in Japanese)
4. ISO 14708–5, Implants for surgery — Active implantable medical devices — Part 5: Circulatory support devices, 2010-02-01

# Chapter 8
# Enhancement of Hemocompatibility

## 8.1 What Kinds of Hemocompatibility Should be Considered

Fundamental problems of hemocompatibility in the development of VADs are hemolysis, thrombus formation, and von Willebrand factor (vWF) damage (Fig. 8.1).

## 8.2 What Is Hemolysis and Its Criterion

Hemolysis, or blood cell damage, is a phenomenon in which the hemoglobin leaks out from erythrocytes, namely red blood cells, to plasma. The causes are due to mechanical fracture, difference of permeability, or some disease.

Mechanical fracture of blood was investigated, and Hashimoto et al. [1] found using cone rheometer that hemolysis occurs for high shear stress and for long exposure time, which is similar to S-N curve for mechanical fatigue (Figs. 8.2 and 8.3).

Among them Giersiepen et al. [2] derived an empirical equation for hemolysis as follows (Fig. 8.4):

$$\frac{\Delta Hb}{Hb}(\%) = 3.62 \times 10^{-5} {t_e}^{0.785} \tau^{2.416}$$

where ΔHb, plasma free hemoglobin; $t_e$, exposure time (ms), and τ, shear stress (Pa).

Comparing animal tests and flow visualization, Nishida et al. [3] obtained empirical threshold as 300 Pa (100,000 $s^{-1}$) for hemolysis (NIH = 0.01) in a blood pump (Fig. 8.4). Nevaril et al. [4] found minimum hemolysis level as



T. Yamane, *Mechanism of Artificial Heart*, DOI 10.1007/978-4-431-55831-6_8

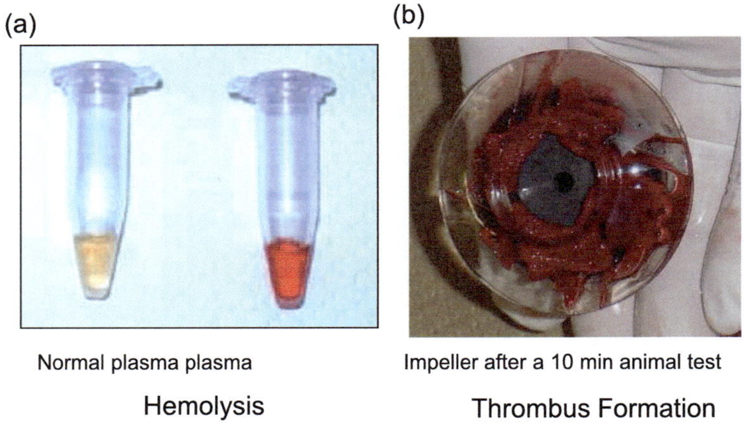


**Fig. 8.1** Hemolysis and thrombus formation observed in a centrifugal blood pump

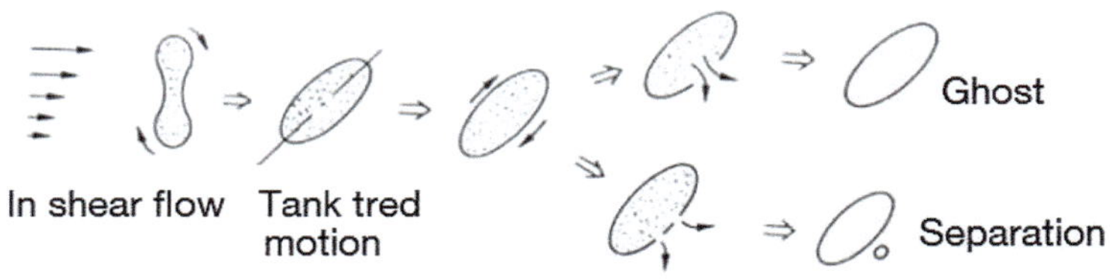


**Fig. 8.2** Mechanism of hemolysis – fatigue of cells [1]

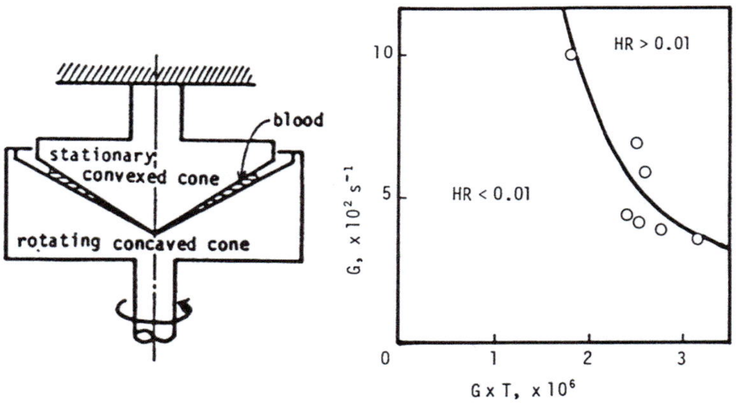


**Fig. 8.3** Effect of shear rate and exposure time on hemolysis. A curve shows iso-hemolysis rate (HR) curve [1]

200 Pa (70,000 $s^{-1}$), and Schima [5] found maximum allowable hemolysis level as 1000 Pa (300,000 $s^{-1}$). These values are almost consistent with one another.

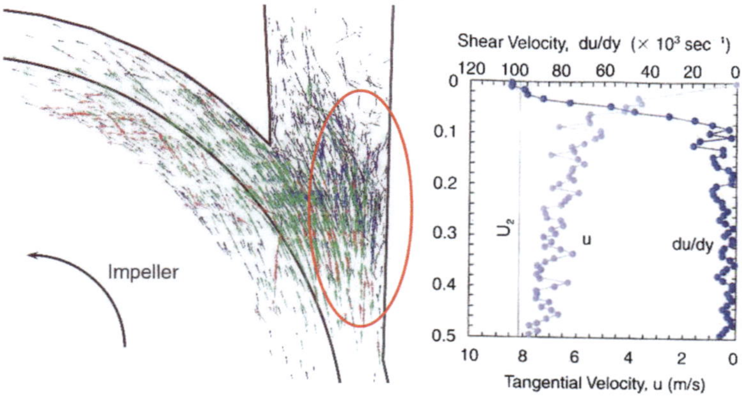


**Fig. 8.4** Effect of shear stress at hemolysis region [3]

It was also experimentally suggested that not only the fluid dynamic friction but also solid wall friction affects hemolysis, especially at pivot bearing as was described in the chapter of pivot bearing.

## 8.3 What Is Thrombus Formation and Its Criterion

Thrombus formation, or blood coagulation, is a blood response to external substances.

Though there are many chains of thrombus formation as is shown in Fig. 8.5, typical processes can be classified by International Standard, ISO 10993–4, [6] to following categories:

1. Coagulation cascade system: Fibrinogen in blood changes to fibrin network under the existence of thrombin. This can be regarded as being triggered rather by molecular-scale chemical signals. And the network collects red blood cells to form a deposition, which is often called as red thrombus.
2. Platelet system: Platelets are activated to extend "legs" on a surface of external materials or damaged blood vessels. This can be regarded as being triggered rather by cell-scale physical signals. The clot is often called as white thrombus.
3. Complement system: Leukocyte activation promotes thrombus formation, which is often called as white thrombus also.

The empirical threshold for thrombus contours is reported as 100 $s^{-1}$ for coagulation by Hashimoto and 300 $s^{-1}$ for red thrombus deposition (Fig. 8.6) or 1700 $s^{-1}$ for white thrombus deposition (Fig. 8.7) by Yamane et al.

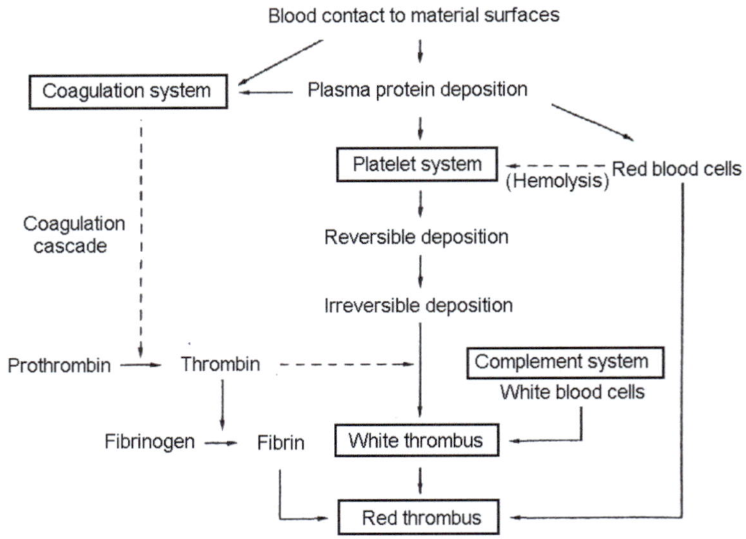


**Fig. 8.5** Mechanism of thrombus formation – coagulation cascade, platelets, and complement systems (Courtesy of Dr. Kozaburo Hayashi)

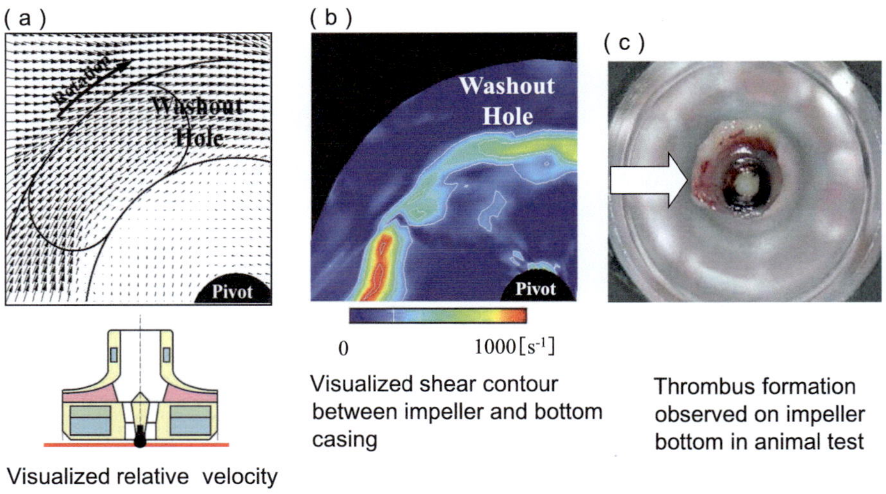


**Fig. 8.6** Comparison of thrombus formation area between animal test and flow visualization (1) Thrombus corresponds area under 300 $s^{-1}$ [7, 8]

## 8.4 What Is vWF Damage

Recently there have been reported a significant number of rotary VAD patients diagnosed as von Willebrand syndrome or bleeding due to blood damage. This disease is characterized by uncontrollable bleeding due to a decrease in the blood

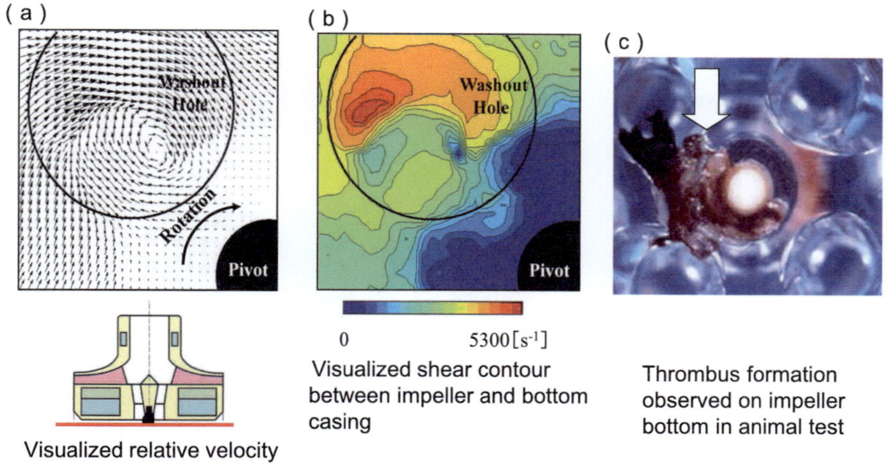


**Fig. 8.7** Comparison of thrombus formation area between animal test and flow visualization (2) Thrombus corresponds area under 1700 $s^{-1}$ [7, 8]

concentration of von Willebrand factor (vWF), a protein in the clotting cascade. Though the relation between rotary VAD and von Willebrand syndrome has not been well investigated yet, a certain lack of molecular weight of vWF and an increase of the lack was recognized, as is denoted by red circles in Fig. 8.8, for patients suffering from bleeding.

Some researchers propose the empirical thresholds for vWF damage is 9 Pa, platelet activation 50 Pa, and hemolysis 150 Pa in stress expression.

## 8.5 Testing Methods

Testing methods of hemocompatibility are proposed for ventricular assist devices, surgical blood pumps, or blood contacting materials. Some of them have been standardized.

### *8.5.1 In Vitro Hemolysis Testing*

A hemolysis testing method for a ventricular assist device is authorized in ASTM F-1841-97 [10]. Regarding the selection of test, blood is precisely written in ASTM F-1830-97 [11]. It says that "blood" should be collected from human or animal, adding anticoagulant, and should be used within 48 h. The hematocrit should be adjusted within $30 \pm 2$ %. ASTM F-1841-97 [10] says that a still blood is compared as a control. "Test loop" should contain $450 \pm 45$ mL blood. Among "pump conditions" flow rate should be kept at $5 \pm 0.25$ L/min and the temperature of the

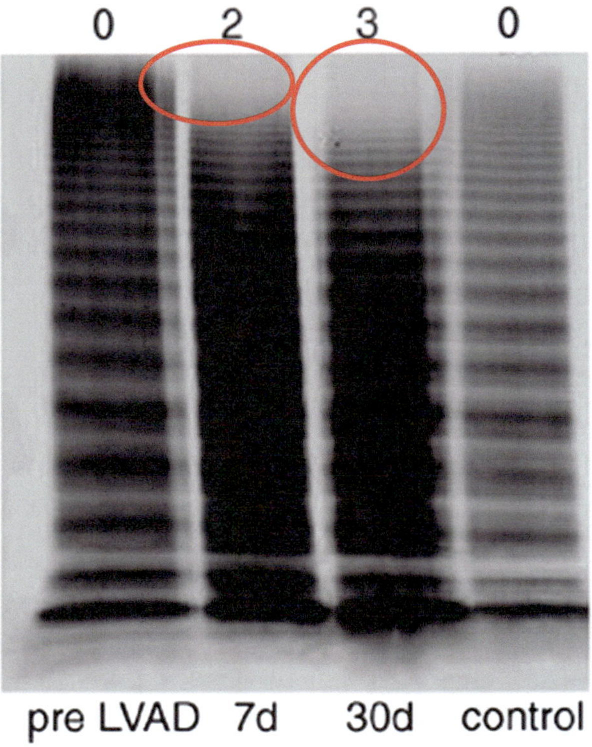


**Fig. 8.8** Damage of von Willebrand factor [9] (Reproduced with permission of Elsevier)

water bath at $37 \pm 1$ °C, and the test should be conducted for 6 h. "Evaluation" is conducted by collecting 1 mL of blood for a sampling and be centrifuged to separate a hemolyzed plasma. This method is a stand-alone testing method without comparison to other devices.

The normalized index of hemolysis (*NIH*) is defined for pumping 100 L blood with $5 \pm 0.25$ L/min flow rate as

$$NIH(g/100L) = \Delta\text{free}Hb \times V \times \frac{100 - Ht}{100} \times \frac{100}{Q \times T}$$
$$unit: \Delta\text{free}Hb(g/L),\ \ V(L),\ \ Ht(\%),\ \ Q(L/\text{min}),\ \ T(\text{min})$$

In the definition of *NIH*, the hemoglobin increment per unit time, $\Delta\text{free}Hb \times V/T$, can be regarded as a characteristic value for the device hemolysis. $(100 - Ht)/100$ is a correction factor from plasma to whole blood and 100/$Q$ can be regarded as a period of 20 min, if the total driven blood volume is 100 L and the flow rate $Q$ is 5 L/min.

Therefore, the author proposes an extended index of hemolysis for tests other than a flow rate of 5 L/min as

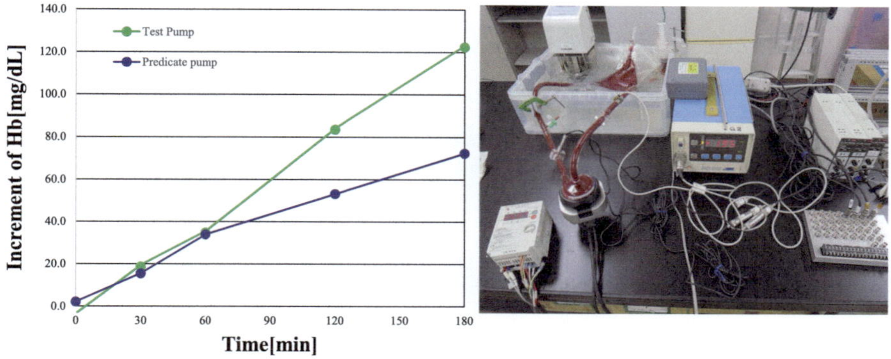


**Fig. 8.9** An example of hemolysis testing

$$NIH(g/20\text{min}) = \Delta\text{free}\,Hb \times V \times \frac{100 - Ht}{100} \times \frac{20}{T}$$
$$unit : \Delta\text{free}\ Hb(g/L),\ \ V(L),\ \ Ht(\%),\ \ T(\text{min})$$

This definition can be applied even for low flow tests or different flow tests.

A relative testing method for surgical blood pumps will be authorized in ISO/CD 18242, [12] under development, "Cardiovascular implants and extracorporeal systems — Centrifugal blood pumps". A commercial pump is compared to a predicate pump, namely pre-evaluated pump. This can compensate the difference of the collected blood quality and the circuit materials (Fig. 8.9).

On the other hand, a testing method regarding contacting materials is authorized in ISO 10993-4, [13].

### 8.5.2 *In Vitro Anti-throbogenicity Testing*

An in vitro testing method of blood coagulation in a pump is proposed before animal testing by Maruyama [14]. A test pump is located in a closed circuit filled with 37°C bovine blood containing trisodium citrate to prevent coagulation. When calcium chloride ($CaCl_2$) is added to the blood for trisodium citrate to have a final concentration of 0.080 w/v%, the blood throbogenicity revives. The activated clotting time (ACT) is kept between 180 and 200 s for around 2 h by adding trisodium citrate to suppress coagulation and by adding calcium chloride to promote coagulation. After two hours, the test device is opened and is observed its thrombus formation.

Figure 8.10 shows an example to compare the thrombus formations before and after the improvement of production accuracy of a pivot geometry.

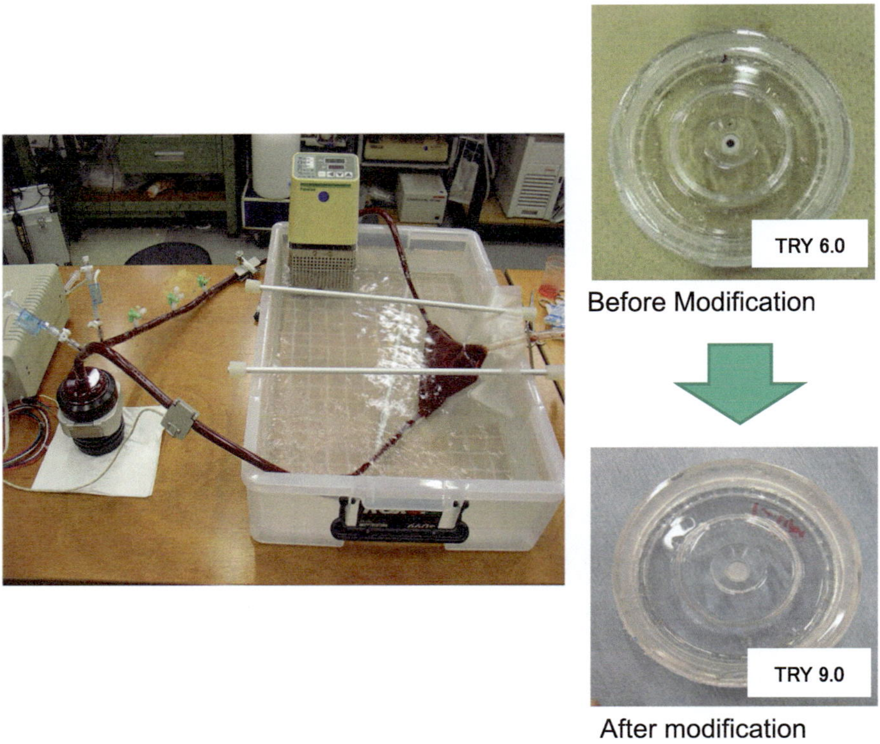


**Fig. 8.10** In vitro anti-throbogenicity testing [14]

## *8.5.3 Animal Testing (In Vivo Evaluation)*

Based on ISO 14708-5 [15], the objective of an animal study is to perform a non-clinical validation of the final device by obtaining safety and performance data in a living animal. The purpose is to evaluate biocompatibility of the device in an appropriate animal model. Safety shall be assessed based on thrombogenicity, hemolysis, calcification, end organ dysfunction, infection, corrosion, hermetic integrity, wear, and other biocompatibility evaluations compared to clinically acceptable limits.

In selection of animal species the body weight, blood cell size or coagulation characteristics are to be considered. The average sizes of erythrocytes, namely red blood cells, are listed in the following table (Table 8.1).

Cow, sheep, or goat are usually used for animal experiments because they do not remove attached medical devices.

**Table 8.1** Comparison of sizes of erythrocytes, namely red blood cells [16]

| Species | μm |
|---|---|
| Human | 8.4 |
| Dog | 7.0 |
| Pig | 6.0 |
| Cat | 5.8 |
| Horse | 5.7 |
| Cow | 5.5 |
| Sheep | 4.5 |
| Goat | 3.2 |

Reproduced with permission of Wiley

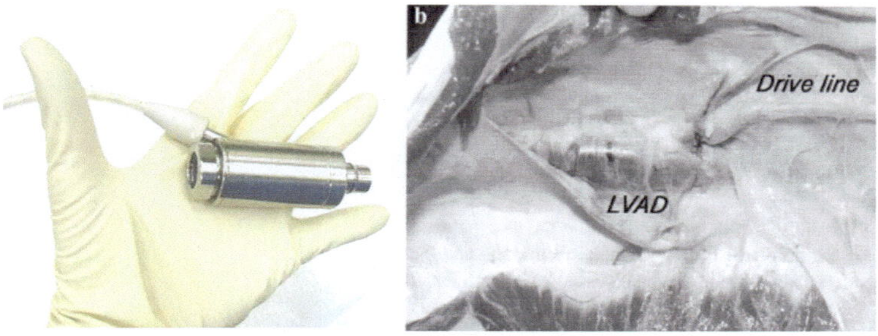


**Fig. 8.11** Animal testing for an axial-flow VAD in eight animals for 90 days [17] (Reproduced with permission of NEDO and National Cerebral and Cardiovascular Center)

Japanese guidance for ventricular assist devices/total artificial hearts, which is compatible to ISO 14708-5, is also applicable to Japanese application for approval. For example, animal testing was conducted for 90 days with eight cows of 60–100 kg body weight regarding an axial-flow VAD developed in NEDO project (Fig. 8.11). In another case for a monopivot centrifugal pump, an animal testing was conducted with goat to improve hemocompatibility (Fig. 8.12).

Practically the animal body weight is selected almost the same as a human because the total blood volume should be similar to a human. A way of tube connection is, for example, extracting from left apex and sending to descending aorta. Heparin, as anticoagulant, can be introduced in an acute stage to keep the activated clotting time, ACT, within 180–200 s or the activated partial thromboplastin time, APTT, within 45–50 s. In a chronic stage it may be switched to warfarin to keep the prothrombin time-international normalized ratio, PT-INR, within 2–3 just like human patients. While anticoagulant is not necessary for heparinized pumps/circuits.

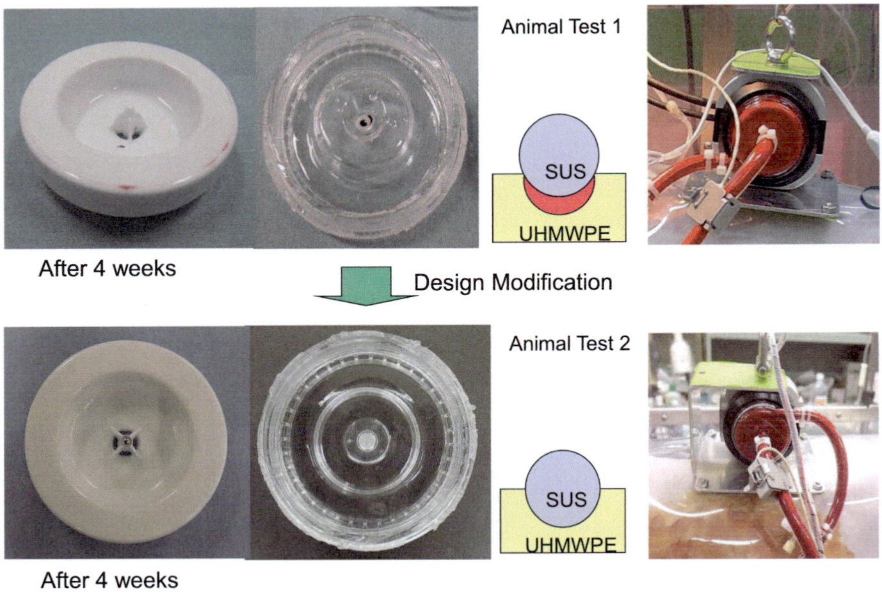


**Fig. 8.12** Animal testing for a surgical centrifugal pump [18]

## References

1. Hashimoto, S.: Erythrocyte destruction under periodically fluctuating shear rate: comparative study with constant shear rate. J. Artif. Organs **13**(5), 458–463 (1989). Blackwell
2. Giersiepen, M., Wurzinger, L.J., Opitz, R., Reul, H.: Estimation of shear stress-related blood damaga in heart valve prostheses-in vitro comparison of 25 aortic valves. Int. J. Artif. Organs **13**(5), 300–306 (1990)
3. Nishida, M., Yamane, T., Masuzawa, T., Tsukiya, T., Taenaka, Y., Tsukamoto, Y., Ito, K., Konishi, Y.: Flow visualization study to obtain suitable design criteria of a centrifugal blood pump. J. Congest. Heart Fail. Circulat. Support **1**(4), 311–315 (2001)
4. Nevaril, C.G., Hellums, J.D., Alfrey Jr., C.P., Lynch, E.C.: Physical effects in red blood cell trauma. A.I.Ch.E. J. **15**, 707 (1969)
5. Schima, H., Wieselthaler, G., Schwendenwein, I., Losert, U., Wolner, E.: A review and assessment of investigative methods for mechanically induced blood trauma: special aspects in rotary blood pumps. Heart Replace Artif. Heart **6**, 361–367 (1998)
6. ISO 10993–4 Biological evaluation of medical devices — Part 4: Selection of tests for interactions with blood
7. Toyoda, M., Nishida, M., Maruyama, O., Yamane, T., Tsutsui, T., Sankai, Y.: Geometric optimization for non-thrombogenicity of a centrifugal blood pump through flow visualization. JSME Int. J. C **45**(4), 1013–1019 (2002)
8. Yamane, T., Maruyama, O., Nishida, M., Toyoda, M., Tsutsui, T., Jikuya, T., Shigeta, O., Sankai, Y.: The most profitable use of flow visualization in the elimination of thrombus from a monopivot magnetic suspension blood pump. J. Artif Organs **28**(4), 390–397 (2004). Blackwell
9. Crow, S., Chen, D., Milano, C., Thomas, W., Joyce, L., Piacentino III, V., Sharma, R., Wu, J., Arepally, G., Bowles, D., Rogers, J., Villamizar-Ortiz, N.: Acquired von Willebrand syndrome

in continuous-flow ventricular assist device recipients. Ann. Thorac. Surg. **90**, 1263–1269 (2010)
10. ASTM F-1830-97, Standard practice for selection of blood for in-vitro evaluation of blood pumps (1997)
11. ASTM F1841-97, Standard practice for Assessment of hemolysis in continuous flow blood pumps (1997)
12. ISO/CD 18242, Cardiovascular implants and extracorporeal systems — Centrifugal blood pumps
13. ISO 10993–4, Biological evaluation of medical devices — Part 4: Selection of tests for interactions with blood, 2013-01-10
14. Maruyama, O., Tomari, Y., Sugiyama, D., Nishida, M., Tsustui, T., Yamane, T.: Simple in vitro testing method for antithrombogenic evaluation of centrifugal blood pumps. ASAIO J. **55**(4), 314–322 (2009)
15. ISO 14708–5, Implants for surgery — Active implantable medical devices — Part 5: Circulatory support devices, 2010-02-01
16. Thrall, M.A., Weiser, G., Allison, R.W., Campbell, T.W.: Veterinary Hematology and Clinical Chemistry, 2nd edn. Wiley-Blackwell, Somerset (2012)
17. Tanaka, H., Tsukiya, T., Tatsumi, E., Mizuno, T., Hidaka, T., Okubo, T., Osada, T., Miyamoto, S., Taenaka, Y.: Initial in vivo evaluation of the newly developed axial flow turbo pump with hydrodynamic bearings. J. Artif. Organs **14**(1), 31–38 (2011). Springer
18. Yamane, T., Kosaka, R., Nishida, M., Maruyama, O., Yamamoto, Y., Kuwana, K., Kawamura, H., Shiraishi, Y., Yambe, T., Sankai, Y., Tsutsui, T.: Enhancement of hemocompatibility of the MERA monopivot centrifugal pump: toward medium-term use. J. Artif. Organs **37**(2), 217–225 (2013). Wiley-Blackwell

# Chapter 9
# System Evaluation

## 9.1 Clinical Trial

First, it would be necessary to explain how VADs are implanted to human body (Fig. 9.1). There are several ways to implant VADs. For recent rotary VADs, blood is extracted from the apex of left ventricle, whose systole pressure is the highest and is sent to ascending aorta or to descending aorta. Sending to ascending aorta means sending blood before the bifurcation to cerebral artery, and sending to descending aorta after the bifurcation. The latter operation is easier since it needs to open only left chest if the blood pump is sufficiently small. Figure 9.2 shows the two operation patterns, for example, of Jarvik 2000.

A brand-new medical device should be evaluated for a full set system in clinical trials, if their safety and efficacy are not well known only by lab tests and documentations. In a case of medical devices, the safety and the efficacy should be evaluated for not only device itself but also how to use the devices. A clinical study is also important before and after the approval.

A ventricular assist device was recognized as a therapy only after a clinical study, the Randomized Evaluation of Mechanical Assistance for the Treatment of Congestive Heart Failure (REMATCH study), 1998–2001, as shown in Fig. 9.3. The clinical study evaluated the suitability of implantable LVADs for the ultimate intended use as a long-term myocardial-replacement therapy. Sixty-eight LVAD patients and sixty-one medical therapy patients were observed who were all ineligible for cardiac transplantation. The result was typically shown in Kaplan–Meier survival analysis as the one-year survival rates of 52 % for LVAD assist and 25 % for medical therapy. The result showed a typical scientific evidence for LVAD therapy.

The survival rates of VADs are now much improved as Fig. 9.4.



T. Yamane, *Mechanism of Artificial Heart*, DOI 10.1007/978-4-431-55831-6_9

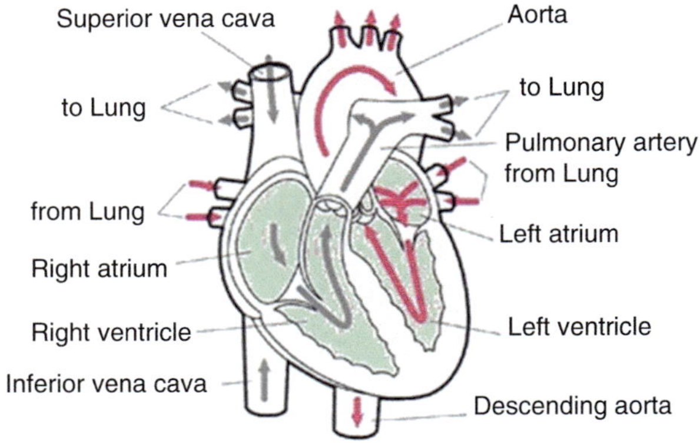


**Fig. 9.1** Human circulation around heart

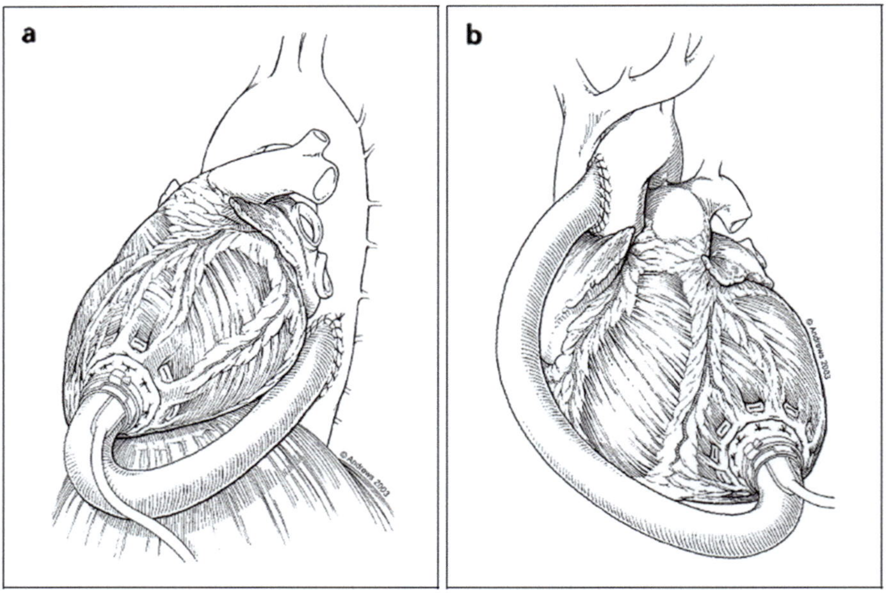


**Fig. 9.2** Two ways of implantation of a VAD, an example of Jarvik 2000 [1] (Reproduced with permission of S. Karger AG)

## 9.2 Regulatory Science

### *9.2.1 Standard and Guidance*

Most general standard for ventricular assist systems is International Standard, ISO 14708-5 [3]. Items of requirements for particular active implantable medical devices are listed as follows:

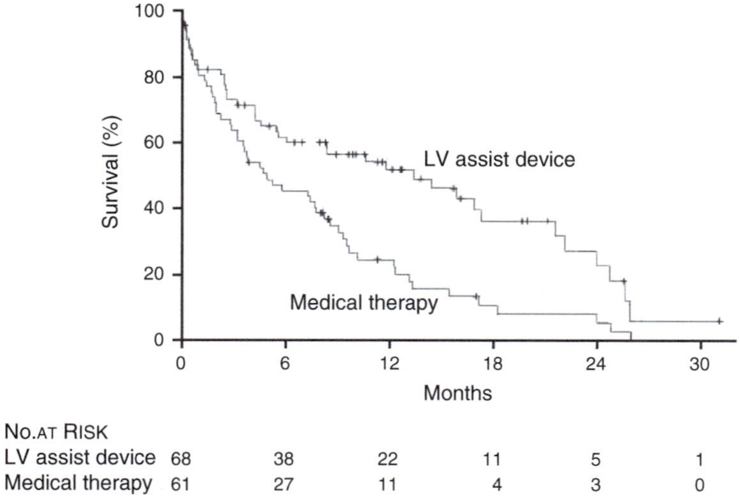


**Fig. 9.3** Randomized Evaluation of Mechanical Assistance for the Treatment of Congestive Heart Failure (REMATCH) clinical study [2]

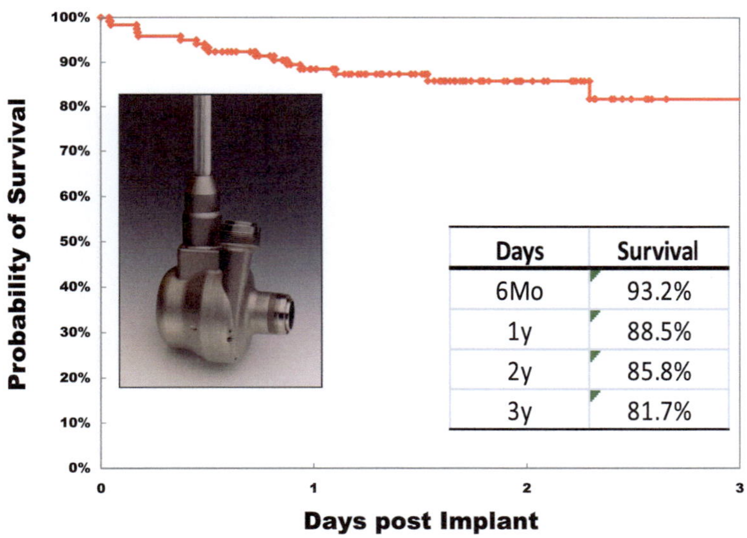


**Fig. 9.4** Survival rate of a recent VAD (a case of EVAHEART; Reproduced with permission of Sun Medical Technology Research Corp. and Tokyo Women's Medical University)

1. Intended clinical use/indications
2. System description
3. Design analysis
4. Risk analysis
5. Human factors

6. In vitro design evaluation and system performance testing
7. Electromagnetic compatibility
8. Materials qualification
9. Biocompatibility
10. Environmental testing
11. In vivo evaluation
12. Reliability
13. Clinical evaluation: see ISO 14155

In Japan from 2005 to 2007 the Ministry of Health, Labor and Welfare (MHLW) and the Ministry of Economy, Trade and Industry (METI) organized working groups mostly from academia to establish Japanese guidance for VAD/TAH. The METI published the R&D Guidelines for innovative artificial hearts in 2007, and the MHLW published a Notification by Director in 2008 regarding the evaluation criteria for emerging technology. Correspondingly,

R&D guidance describes the following items:

1. Purpose of use
2. Human factors and environments
3. Fluid dynamic characteristics
4. Heating characteristics
5. Electronic safety
6. Electro-magnetic compatibility
7. Control and monitoring
8. Conduits, grafts, artificial heart valves, or heart cuff
9. Materials safety
10. Biocompatibility
11. Animal testing
12. Durability (Reliability)

Annex A. Supplement for TAH
Annex B. Supplement for durability test
Annex C. Supplement for out-of-hospital program

Clinical evaluation guidance describes the following items:

1. Fundamentals: Human factors and environments
2. Non-clinical evaluation: In vitro evaluation and in vivo evaluation
3. Clinical evaluation

Annex 1. Durability test (Same as R&D guidance)
Annex 2. Sample size and duration for animal testing (Same as R&D guidance)
Annex 3. Out-of-hospital program (Same as R&D guidance)
Annex 4. Sample size and duration for clinical trials
Annex 5. Facilities for clinical trials
Annex 6. Final evaluation

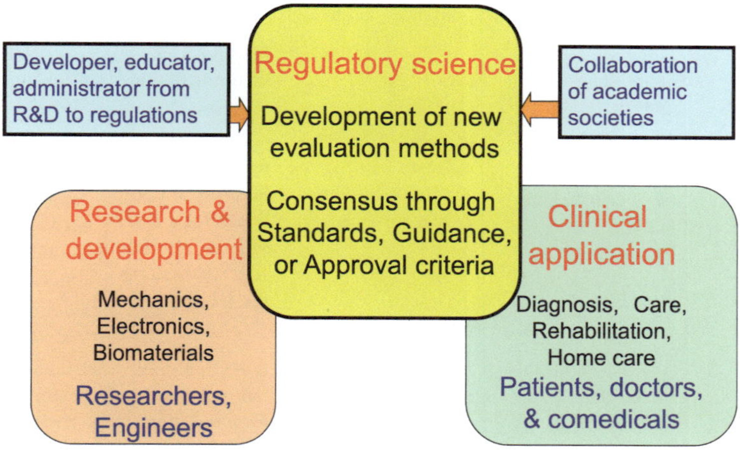


**Fig. 9.5** Concept of regulatory science

They defined minimum evaluation requirements as scientific evidences to the industries and to the government, which enabled industries to develop efficiently and enabled the government to review quickly. Though the guidance is not at all a law or a standard, this indication can be regarded as a typical case for regulatory science. The content includes a little more details than the ISO. After the settlement, more than four kinds of VADs have been approved based on the Japanese guidance.

Figure 9.5 shows the role of regulatory science. Newly developed medical devices by researchers and/or engineers are evaluated through standards, guidance, and/or approval criteria to obtain approval. And then they are handed to patients, doctors, and/or co-medicals.

Table 9.1 shows a detail comparison between historical guidance and standards. Regarding reliability testing, the FDA guidance [4] (1987) requested that X or more devices are used with less than Y failures over twice the intended use for short-term use and over Z years for long-term use. The ASAIO-STS [5] (1998) required 80 % reliability with at least 60 % confidence for 1 year mission life. The NCTIS required the same level before Investigative Device Exemption (IDE). The ISO/DIS requires that a reliability of X with at least Y confidence for a Z-year mission life is described. The Japanese guidance requires 80 % reliability with at least 60 % (80 %) confidence for 6 months, similar to the ASAIO-STS recommendation.

Regarding animal testing, the FDA [4] required a duration of 5 months. The ASAIO-STS [5] reduced the request to eight animals for 90 days before IDE. The ISO/DIS requires only that the sample size and duration are described. The Japanese guidance reduced the request to at least six animals for 60 days with consideration of eight animals for 90 days if necessary, which is a small reduction from the ASAIO-STS recommendation.

Regarding clinical trials, the Japanese guidance [6–8] referred to practical goals for a feasibility study and for a pivotal study, although most guidance documents

**Table 9.1** Comparison of historical guidance documents and standards for VAD/TAH [8]

| | Japanese guidelines (2007–2008) | ISO 14708-5 (2010) | ASAIO-STS recommedation (1998) | FDA guidelines (1987) |
|---|---|---|---|---|
| Reliability test (in vitro) | **80 %** reliability, | Reliability **X** with at least **Y** confidence for a **Z** year mission life | A calculated **80 %** reliability with at least **60 %** confidence for a **1 year** mission life Before IDE ≧8 systems for ≧1 year | ≧**X** devices with ≦**Y** failures |
| | **60 % (80 %)** confidence, and **6 months** (to be extended≧2 years) | | | ***Short term***: over ≧**twice** the intended duration |
| | | | | ***Lomg term***: over ≧**Z years** |
| Animal test (in vivo) | At least **6 animals for 60 days** (8 animals for 90 days) | Sample size and implant duration to demonstrate the safety and performance for the intended use | IDE: In a minimum of **8 animals** for a duration ≧**90 days** | Durability and performance for ≧**twice** the expected duration |
| | | | | Permanent implant device for ≧**5 months** |
| Clinical trial | Sample size: Around **15** cases for a pivotal study (Around 5 cases for a feasibility study) | ISO 14155-1 and ISO 14155-2 | PMA: All in vitro, in vivo, and clinical data reported by category: The number of patients and the number of patient-years | A rationale for the number of patients and institutions required to the safety and efficacy |
| | *End point:* **6 months** for BTT, and **12 (&24) months** for DT as a pivotal study (3 months as a feasibility study) | | | (Preliminary IDE study: 5–10 patients at 1–2 centers) |

and standards do not refer to practical periods. The present guidance is expected to contribute to the approval of VAD/TAH in Japan.

A recent topic of regulatory science is a topic of destination therapy (DT). DT does not only mean a permanent use of VADs but also means a release of restrictions to patient selection criteria such as age, pulmonary function, renal function, hepatic function, etc. Which item should be released to what extent are the argument points. Regarding the age, elderly patients lose opportunities for VAD application. Pediatric patients with intrinsic diseases have problems for the following transplantation. These are ethical and economical problems.

# References


1. Frazier, O.H., Shah, N.A., Myers, T.J., Robertson, K.D., Gregoric, I.D., Delgado, R.: Use of the flowmaker (Jarvik 2000) left ventricular assist device for destination therapy and bridging to transplantation. Cardiology **101**, 111–116 (2004)
2. Rose, E.A., Gelijns, A.C., Moskowitz, A.J., Heitjan, D.F., Stevenson, L.W., Dembitsky, W., Long, J.W., Ascheim, D.D., Tierney, A.R., Levitan, R.G., Watson, J.T., Meier, P.: Long term use of a left ventricular assist device for end stage heart failure. N. Engl. J. Med. **345**(20), 1435–1443 (2001)
3. ISO 14708-5, Implants for surgery — Active implantable medical devices — Part 5: Circulatory support devices, 2010-02-01
4. FDA: Preparation and contents of application for ventricular assist devices and total artificial hearts, FDA No. F89-33838 (1987)
5. ASAIO-STS: Long-Term Mechanical Circulatory Support System Reliability Recommendation (1998)
6. METI, Japan. R&D Guidlines for active implants 2007: Innovative artificial heart systems, May 2007. Available at: http://www.meti.go.jp/policy/mono_info_service/healthcare/report_iryou_fukushi.html
7. MHLW, Japan. Notification by Director, OMDE, Yakushokuki-hatsu No. 0404002: Evaluation criteria for emerging technology: Clinical evaluation criteria for next-generation artificial hearts, April 4, (2008). Available at: http://dmd.nihs.go.jp/jisedai/heart/heart_public.pdf
8. Yamane, T., Kyo, S., Matsuda, H., Abe, Y., Imachi, K., Masuzawa, T., Nakatani, T., Sase, K., Tabayashi, K., Takatani, S., Tatsumi, E., Umezu, M., Tsuchiya, T.: Japanese guidance for ventricular assist devices/total artificial hearts. J. Artif. Organs **34**(9), 699–702 (2010). Wiley-Blackwell

# Chapter 10
# Remarks and Future Aspect

Artificial hearts, most of them are ventricular assist devices, developed from hospital use to home care during around 60 years. Rotary pumps reduced the size of pulsatile pumps to be portable or implantable. Rotary pumps also enabled us to implement high-durability bearings, which allowed patients to go out of hospital. The longest patient lives nearly 10 years with the implantable VAD. These developments have been realized historically by the collaboration between a medical team, an engineering team, and an administrative team.



T. Yamane, *Mechanism of Artificial Heart*, DOI 10.1007/978-4-431-55831-6_10

MIX
Papier aus verantwortungsvollen Quellen
Paper from responsible sources
FSC® C105338

If you have any concerns about our products,
you can contact us on
**ProductSafety@springernature.com**

In case Publisher is established outside the EU,
the EU authorized representative is:
**Springer Nature Customer Service Center GmbH**
**Europaplatz 3, 69115 Heidelberg, Germany**

Printed by Libri Plureos GmbH
in Hamburg, Germany